deep humility. ‘

‘The interweaving of a historical perspective is a highlight of the narrative and adds a richness that makes *Shapeshifters* such a pleasure to read.’ *Lancet*

‘Such is the breadth of Francis’ interests that *Shapeshifters* is never less than intellectually energetic.’ Brian Dillon, *Guardian*

‘[An] enthralling collection of illustrated pieces about human transformation … Francis will leave you marvelling at the physical self you carry around with you every day.’ *Sunday Express*

‘A thoughtful exploration … Francis’ wide-ranging experience and curiosity produce fascinating samples of medical and cultural approaches to human change.’ *Publishers Weekly*

‘Gavin Francis makes being a doctor sound like the best job in the world … The essays in this collection … all circle the theme of metamorphosis, and shed light on the biases of modern medicine even while celebrating its achievements.’ *Village Voice*

‘What makes the book fun to read is not only the author’s limpid anecdotes from his private practice, but also his abiding marvel at the body’s endless expressions. Francis ranges freely and skilfully from the strange to the elemental … [he] always makes you think.’ *Kirkus Reviews*

‘As compelling as it is affecting’ *Scotland on Sunday*

GAVIN FRANCIS is a doctor and writer. He is the author of *Adventures in Human Being*, which won the Saltire Non-Fiction Book of the Year, as well as *True North* and *Empire Antarctica*, which won the Scottish Book of the Year Award and was shortlisted for both the Ondaatje Prize and Costa Prize. He also writes for the *Guardian*, *The Times*, *London Review of Books* and *Granta*. He lives and practises medicine in Edinburgh, where he's a member of the Royal College of Emergency Medicine and a Fellow of the Royal College of General Practitioners.

Find him on Twitter *@gavinfranc*

And online at *www.gavinfrancis.com*

SHAPESHIFTERS

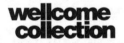

WELLCOME COLLECTION is a free museum and library that aims to challenge how we think and feel about health. Inspired by the medical objects and curiosities collected by Henry Wellcome, it connects science, medicine, life and art. Wellcome Collection exhibitions, events and books explore a diverse range of subjects, including consciousness, forensic medicine, emotions, sexology, identity and death.

Wellcome Collection is part of Wellcome, a global charitable foundation that exists to improve health for everyone by helping great ideas to thrive, funding over 14,000 researchers and projects in more than seventy countries.

wellcomecollection.org

SHAPESHIFTERS

A Doctor's Notes on
Medicine & Human Change

GAVIN FRANCIS

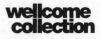

This paperback edition published in 2019

First published in Great Britain in 2018 by
Profile Books Ltd
3 Holford Yard
Bevin Way
London
WC1X 9HD
www.profilebooks.com

Published in association with Wellcome Collection

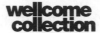

183 Euston Road
London NW1 2BE
www.wellcomecollection.org

1 3 5 7 9 10 8 6 4 2

Typeset in Sabon by MacGuru Ltd
Printed and bound in Great Britain by
CPI Group (UK) Ltd, Croydon CR0 4YY

A CIP catalogue record for this book is
available from the British Library.

ISBN 978 1 78125 774 6
eISBN 978 1 78283 323 9
Export ISBN 978 1 78816 141 1

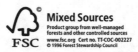

Mixed Sources
Product group from well-managed
forests and other controlled sources
www.fsc.org Cert no. TT-COC-002227
© 1996 Forest Stewardship Council

For life's optimists,
who see hope in human change

LECTOR INTENDE, LAETABERIS

Mankind –
N. human race, human species, human kind, human
  nature; humanity.
  human being; person, individual, mortal, body.

Adj. human, mortal, personal, individual, social.

Change –
N. alteration, mutation, variation, modification,
  metastasis, deviation, turn, evolution, revolution,
    transformation, transfiguration; metamorphosis.

V. alter, vary; modulate, turn, shift, veer, shuffle, swerve,
  deviate.
    transform, transfigure, metamorphose.

My aim is to sing of the ways bodies change, ceaselessly transforming into other forms.

Ovid, *Metamorphoses* (c. 8 CE)

All things change with time, and we change with them.

Lothar, Holy Roman Emperor (c. 840)

And then I, a woman, by a flick of Fortune's hand was transformed into a man.

Christine de Pizan, *The Mutation of Fortune* (1403)

We are nothing but a bundle or collection of different sensations ... and are in a perpetual flux and movement.

David Hume, *A Treatise of Human Nature* (1739)

It is itself unchanged, the same water which my youthful eyes fell on; all the change is in me.

Henry David Thoreau, *Walden* (1854)

Metamorphosis governs natural phenomena ... reflects the shifting character of knowledge and attitudes to the human.

Marina Warner, *Ovidian Metamorphosis in Contemporary Art* (2009)

Contents

A note on confidentiality

THIS BOOK IS A SERIES OF STORIES about medicine and the changing human body. Just as physicians must honour the privileged access they have to our bodies, they must honour the trust with which we share our stories. Even as long as two and a half thousand years ago that obligation was recognised: the Hippocratic Oath insists 'whatsoever in the course of practice you see or hear that ought never to be published abroad, you will not divulge'. As a doctor who is also a writer I've spent a great deal of time deliberating over that use of 'ought', considering what can and cannot be said without betraying the confidence of my patients.

The reflections that follow are all grounded in events within my clinical experience, but the patients in them have been so disguised as to be unrecognisable — any similarities that remain are coincidental. Protecting confidences is an essential part of what I do: 'confidence' means 'with faith' – we are all patients sooner or later; we all want faith that we'll be heard, and that our privacy will be respected.

1

Transformation

From so simple a beginning endless forms most beautiful and most wonderful have been, and are being, evolved.

Charles Darwin, *On the Origin of Species*

THERE'S A PARK near my medical office lined with cherry trees and elms that undergo beautiful annual transformations. If there's time on my commute I'll stop at a bench and watch them for a few moments. Winter brings storms, and the last few years have seen several of the tallest elms blown over. When they fall down, tearing up their roots, deep coffin-sized gashes open in the earth. Around Easter the branches thicken with a green so enchanting I see why some imagine it as the colour of heaven. The blossoming of the cherry trees in spring strews the grass with petals, and to take a stroll beneath their branches is to be fêted in pink. The summer air feels ripe and dense – barbecues are lit and babies play on rugs in the shade; acrobats teeter over ropes strung between the tree trunks. But my favourite season is autumn, when the sky feels high, the air pellucid and brittle, and heaps of crimson, auburn and gold gather around my feet. I've been appreciating this park for around twenty-five years – it's adjacent to the medical school where I trained.

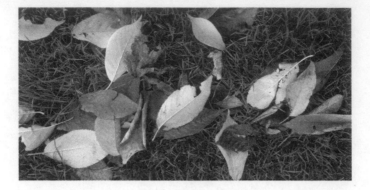

Aged eighteen, in the first year of training, I walked through drifts of those leaves to a biochemistry class that I've never forgotten – a lecture where I had something approaching a revelation of the intricacy, the intercon- nectedness, even the wonder of life. It had an inauspicious beginning: projected on the wall was a complex diagram of the haemoglobin molecule. The tutor explained that the chemical which binds oxygen into red blood cells, known as a 'porphyrin ring', was essential both to the haemoglobin of blood and the chlorophyll that traps the sun's energy in leaves. Thanks to porphyrins, she said, life on earth as we know it is possible. Up on the wall, the molecular struc- ture resembled a four-leafed clover, with porphyrin leaves interlocked in an architecture of almost Gothic complexity. Cradled at the core of each of the four leaves was a lava-red atom of iron.

When oxygen binds to the heart of each leaf, she explained, it reddens like an autumn maple; when oxygen is released, it darkens to purple. So far, so biochemical. 'But this isn't a static process,' the tutor added, 'it's dynamic and alive.' The binding of oxygen transforms its cradle; the stress of that transformation pulls a tiny atomic lever which bends the cradles of the other three, encouraging the take-up of more oxygen. The elegance of biochemistry struck me as a revelation, as startling as it should have been obvious: from chlorophyll to haemoglobin, molecules cooperate with one another in order to sustain life.

Watching the diagram, I tried to imagine billions of molecules of my own haemoglobin, their shapes shifting as they gathered oxygen in my lungs with each breath. Then the beating of my heart pushing on rivers of blood to my brain, my muscles, my liver, where the same shift would occur in reverse. It seemed a transformation as vital and as perennial as the annual growth and fall of leaves, implausible, somehow, that it could be happening moment to moment throughout my body.

I felt the air charge with reverence, the unfolding of a kind of joy: that such balance existed among the tumult of body chemistry seemed strangely beautiful, though at the same time inevitable.

TRANSFORMATION IS ONE of the most ancient and resonant themes in literature and art: two thousand years ago in the *Metamorphoses*, the Latin poet Ovid painted nature and mankind as a maelstrom where all matter, animate and inanimate, was caught up in cycles of change 'like pliant wax which, stamped with new designs, does not remain as it was, or keep the same shape ... everything is in a state of flux, and comes into being as a transient appearance'. Ovid closed his poem with a declaration of the fraternity of life, and a passionate plea to treat all beings with compassion. That compassion too is at the heart of clinical practice – medicine could be described as the alliance of science with kindness.

To be alive is to be in perpetual metamorphosis. The borders of our selves are porous – shaped and recomposed by elements of our environment. River water was once sea spray; next year it could flow in your neighbour's blood. The water in your brain once fell as rain on ancient landscapes, and surged in the swell of long-gone oceans.

From this perspective, the body is itself a flowing stream, or burning fire: no two of its moments are ever the same. In growth and in recovery, in adapting and in ageing, our bodies ineludibly change form – and with sleep, memory and learning, so do our minds. On a routine day in my clinic as a general practitioner I see a minimum of twelve patients in the morning, and another twelve in the afternoon; the twenty-four chapters of this book are as eclectic as those twenty-four consultations can be, and look into the ways my work as a physician takes advantage of those changes that aid us, and tries to slow those changes that would constrain us. They examine just a selection of those transformations that, as a doctor, it feels like a privilege to witness.

There's a great deal of overlap between the following categories but about a quarter of the chapters are dedicated to those great transitions of life, when we shift from one phase to another: conception, birth, puberty, pregnancy, menopause, death. More and more we ask our physicians to assist in those transitions. Another quarter of the chapters look at medical crises with the power to change our bodies and minds, such as amputations, fractures, hormonal imbalances, and even cancer. Moment to moment our minds are in constant flux, and about a quarter of the chapters examine those changes that transform our mental experience, from the nightly retreat into sleep, to the fundamental significance of memory, to some of the many different manifestations of mental illness that as a general practitioner I'm asked to alleviate. And a final group of chapters examine those changes we decide to impose on the body through an act of will; we can choose to build up our muscles, tattoo, enhance, or in other ways re-sculpt our bodies, either to fit an ideal, or to more closely align with what we see as our authentic selves. My work as a doctor seeks to facilitate those changes where they're helpful, and mitigate those that might be harmful.

The word 'patient' means 'sufferer', and to practise medicine is to seek to ease human suffering. As a writer, I'm interested in change as a metaphor that has preoccupied poets, artists and thinkers for millennia, and as a doctor, I'm interested in the same theme because to practise medicine is to seek positive change, however modest, in the minds and the bodies of my patients. I'd like this book to be read as a celebration of dynamism and transformation in human life, both as a way of thinking about the body, and as a universal truth. That change is not only possible, but inevitable, is a message that offers hope.

2

Werewolves: Agitation at the Full Moon

As the first human metamorphosis of its kind, Lycaon's transformation [into a wolf] is worth examining in detail.

Genevieve Liveley, *Ovid's 'Metamorphoses'*

WHEN A NIGHT in the emergency department is particularly blood-soaked with violence, or heavy with psychiatric admissions, it's common to hear colleagues remark: 'It must be a full moon.' On a busy night shift I've even stepped outside to check, seeking explanation in the heavens for my busy workload on earth. That the moon has effects not just on the tides or on cycles of human fertility, but on minds, is an ancient belief. Othello says to Emilia, 'It is the very error of the moon. She comes more near the earth than she was wont and makes men mad.' James Joyce in *Ulysses* waxes on the moon's 'power to enamour, to mortify, to invest with beauty, to render insane'. That the moon has a transformative effect on the human psyche is a widespread conviction – a variety of studies from India, Iran, Europe and the US have all asserted it. One North American study found that 40 per cent of the general public were convinced that the moon had an influence on the mind; an earlier survey put the rate for mental health professionals at 74 per cent. But statisticians haven't been able to substantiate the claim: the number of admissions for trauma, or for mania or psychosis ('lunacy'), are unaffected by the phase of the moon, and there is no connection between a full moon and the frequency of suicide attempts, road accidents or calls to crisis support telephone services. My colleagues in emergency medicine, and those 74 per cent of American mental health professionals, are all wrong.

That the truth runs counter to such a widely held opinion led three Californian psychiatrists to investigate. In a study called 'The Moon and Madness Reconsidered', they proposed that before the advent of effective artificial lighting in the nineteenth century, the full moon probably did affect those with precarious mental health, by disturbing quality and duration of sleep. They cited evidence that resting in the dark for fourteen hours a day can terminate or even prevent episodes of manic psychosis, and that even a mild reduction in hours of sleep can worsen mental health and bring on epileptic seizures – something my own patients with bipolar illness and epilepsy have confirmed. Patterns of activity in the brain involved in healthy sleep seem to overlap with patterns associated with good mental health in ways we don't yet fully understand.

Before artificial lighting, people took advantage of the days around a full moon, because its light was powerful enough to be abroad at night. The Lunar Society of industrialists and intellectuals in eighteenth-century England named itself not for its object of study but because its members found it easier to meet on evenings when the moon was full. But moonlight was also shadowy enough to give a prompt to the fearful imagination. 'The insane are more agitated at the full of the moon, as they are also at early dawn,' the French psychiatrist Jean-Étienne Esquirol wrote in the nineteenth century: 'Does not this brightness produce, in their habitations, an effect of light, which frightens one, rejoices another, and agitates all?'

JOANNE FREDERICK was brought in by ambulance; 'agitated delirium' was written across the top of her triage sheet. The medical history came from her flatmate: she'd been suffering with a head cold for a few days, feeling weak and under the weather, and had gone to the pharmacy to buy medicine. It didn't work: she became weaker, had abdominal pains, and her skin felt as if it was burning. Her urine felt hot and heavy, and was painful to pass. She'd had urine infections in the past, but this was different: a bodily unease had possessed her, spreading up through her torso and out into her limbs. Her legs trembled, her arms lost all their power, and she had a persistent low-grade fever. She arranged an appointment to see her GP, but never made it: her flatmate called an ambulance when she began hallucinating giant lizards on the walls. On the way to hospital in the ambulance she had a seizure and when I met her in the high-dependency unit, she had been sedated.

There are hundreds of reasons that someone might end up with an 'agitated delirium': drug overdoses, drug withdrawal, infections, strokes, brain haemorrhage, head injuries, psychiatric disorders, and even some vitamin deficiencies. But all of Joanne's blood tests came back normal – the CT scan of her brain was unremarkable. As she lay sedated in the high-dependency unit, her flatmate began to tell me more of her story. Joanne lived a fairly quiet life, with a few close friends but keeping largely to herself. She'd been admitted to hospital with a 'nervous breakdown' once before; the hospital notes said that she'd had a brief episode of incapacitating panic and anxiety that had resolved after a few days' rest. She worked as an administrator in the basement of the city council offices – a job she loved because it allowed her to stay out of the sun. 'She burns really easily,' said her flatmate, 'you should see her in the summer – she gets blisters from it.' Her skin was mottled with brown pigments, particularly across the face and hands, as if coffee granules had been spilled over wet skin.

I was a junior doctor at the time, and for me and the rest of the medical team Joanne's diagnosis was a puzzle. When the supervising physician arrived to do his rounds he listened carefully to the story of how Joanne had come to be there, and flicked through the hospital notes from her previous admission. He examined her skin closely, leafed through the reams of normal tests, then looked up with a glance of triumph: '… we need to check her porphyrins,' he said.

Porphyrins, critical for both the structure of haemoglobin and chlorophyll, are generated in the body by a series of specialised enzymes that work together like a team of scaffolders. If one of those scaffolders doesn't work properly, porphyria is the result. Part-formed rings of porphyrin build up in the blood and tissues bringing on 'crises', which can be occasioned by drugs, diet, and even a couple of nights of insomnia. Some porphyrins are exquisitely sensitive to light (it's this property that enables them to absorb the sun's energy in chlorophyll) and some types of porphyria lead to a blistering inflammation on exposure to the sun, with consequent scarring. The build-up of porphyrins in nerves and the brain causes numbness, paralysis, psychosis and seizures. Another effect of the accumulation of porphyrins in the skin, as yet unexplained, is growth of hair on the forehead and cheeks. Acute porphyria can cause constipation and agonising abdominal pain: it's not unusual for victims to be brought howling into operating theatres, subjected to unnecessary operations time and again before doctors reach the correct diagnosis.*

When Joanne's lab report came back it confirmed soaring levels of porphyrins: it was likely that she had a rare variant of porphyria known as 'variegate'. Treatment had already begun: rest, avoidance of exacerbating drugs

---

* When those same scaffolder enzymes fail in plants, dark spots bloom across the leaves following even modest light exposure.

(the cold remedies she'd bought over the counter had probably triggered her crisis) and intravenous fluids. To those we added infusions of glucose. Within three days she had recovered, and was discharged home from the ward with a list of drugs to avoid and an explanation, at last, of why she'd always been sensitive to light.

IN 1964 A CURIOUS PAPER was published in the journal *Proceedings of the Royal Society of Medicine* by a London neurologist called Lee Illis. In four eloquent and persuasive pages he proposed that the myth of werewolves has been reinforced or even initiated by porphyria. Skin conditions such as hypertrichosis may cause hair to grow over the face and hands, but have no psychiatric manifestations. Rabies in humans may induce an agitated, furious state of mind with biting and hallucinations, but without skin changes. Illis pointed out that people with porphyria avoid direct sunlight, and prefer to go about at night. Crises are precipitated by periods of poor sleep or a change in diet. In severe untreated cases sufferers may have pale, yellowish skin caused by jaundice, scarring of the skin, and hair may even begin to grow across their faces. People with certain types of porphyria may suffer derangements in their mental health and become socially isolated, breeding distrust among the wider community.

In past centuries this constellation of symptoms may have attracted accusations of witchcraft. A French exorcist, Henri Boguet, boasted in his *Discours exécrable des Sorciers* (1602) of the number of werewolves and witches he had tortured and put to death: six hundred, including scores of children. 'All these Sorcerers were grievously scratched on the face, arms and legs,' he wrote, 'one of them was so disfigured that he could scarcely be recognised as a human being, nor could anyone look at him without shuddering.' It isn't inconceivable that a light-sensitive, intermittent kind of madness, transposed to an illiterate, isolated, credulous community, could nourish and perpetuate the fear that human beings can transform into wolves. After all, 74 per cent of mental health professionals believe that the full moon can cause madness.

IN ANCIENT HITTITE LAW, to be banished from a community was to be told, 'thou art become a wolf'; we still describe certain excluded people as 'lone wolves'. The first human transformation described in Ovid's *Metamorphoses* is of man into wolf, effected by the gods as retribution for ferocity and cannibalism. Though the threat from wolves has all but disappeared from Europe we still turn to them when we need a metaphor for the predatory or the ravenous: we speak of a 'wolfish grin' and a 'wolfish appetite'; children still tremble at the wolf in the 'Little Red Riding Hood' story, and the one terrorising the Three Little Pigs. Cave paintings of wolves by our palaeolithic ancestors are among the oldest artworks we know of.

'Werewolf' is supposed to refer to the physical transformation of human being into wolf, while the Greek term 'lycanthropy' is now reserved, in English, for the psychiatric delusion that one has become a wolf – a form of psychosis. Psychiatrists have broadened the term's use to take in any delusion that one has been transformed into an animal, but the correct term for that is 'therianthropy' from the Greek *therion* meaning 'beast'. Pliny thought the idea that people could physically turn into wolves absurd, and that it was only the human mind which was capable of transformation: 'That men may be transformed into Wolves and restored again to their former shapes, we must confidently believe to be a loud lie.'

King James I of England (James VI of Scotland) had a particular fascination for the occult, and in his book *Daemonologie* (1597) he wrote of werewolves: 'by the Greekes they were called lykanthropoi which signifieth menwoolfes. But to tell you simplie my opinion ... if anie such thing hath bene, I take it to have proceeded but of a natu-rall super-abundance of Melancholie.' Lycanthropy, then, was thought by King James to be a temporary madness, a psychiatric problem, rather than a physical transformation. The Greek physician Marcellus of Sida agreed: he argued that the werewolves reported to frequent the graveyards of Athens after nightfall were not 'turnskins' – the Roman term for those who could shape-shift into wolves – but deluded. The Byzantine doctor Paul of Aegina wrote that these lycanthropes could be treated with copious bloodlet-ting, sleep, and sedatives – a set of remedies not too different from the modern treatment of porphyria.

Ancient literature is replete with delusional transfor-mations: one of Virgil's *Eclogues* tells of the madness of three sisters, cursed into believing they had become cows: 'They filled the fields with imaginary lowing … each feared the plough-yoke on her neck and often searched for horns on her smooth brow.' In the Bible's Old Testament, King Nebuchadnezzar undergoes an animal transformation fol-lowing a fit of depression: 'He was driven from men, and ate grass as oxen, and his body was wet with the dew of heaven, till his hairs had grown like eagles' feathers, and his nails like birds' claws.'

In late medieval Europe atrocities like those described by Boguet were relatively common: hundreds of would-be werewolves were put to death at the stake. As the eigh-teenth and nineteenth centuries wore on, published reports of 'lycanthropy' began to fade along with superstitions (and European wolf populations). But the delusion didn't go away entirely, it just changed form. In 1954 Carl Jung described three sisters who dreamed night after night that their mother had transformed into an animal. He wasn't surprised when, years later, the mother developed psychotic lycanthropy: the daughters, he reasoned, had unconsciously recognised their mother's long repressed 'primitive identity'.

IN OUR OWN TIMES and culture, the most famous literary work to express the horror and the metaphorical potential of animal transformation is Kafka's *The Metamorphosis*. Gregor Samsa wakes one day as a 'monstrous vermin', an insect-like creature with scurrying legs, horny jaws and a beetle-like shell.* Samsa's transformation is irreversible: as a travelling salesman he was trapped in the service of his family, and in his new life as vermin he is physically trapped in his room. As his family agonise over what to do he gets accustomed to his new form, scuttling on his ceiling, and preferring rotting scraps from the floorboards to the plated food his family leave out for him. In the end he goes the way of all vermin, dead on the floorboards, and swept out with the trash.

Kafka's *Metamorphosis* resists straightforward inter-pretations, but speaks to anyone who feels alienated, persecuted and powerless. Samsa's metamorphosis renders him spatially and socially isolated, like many who suffer profound mental or physical illness. The animal transfor-mations we know of from myth and from folklore traditions tend to carry a semblance of coherence, or even justice, at least within the logic of their own story. But Samsa doesn't have that consolation: 'he could think of no way of bring-ing peace and order to this chaos.'

ONE OF THE ELM TREES near my clinic seems to me different from all the others, not because of its size, or the pattern of its limbs, but because one of my patients once fell twenty feet from it. Gary Hobbes wasn't normally a tree-climber: he was a young man with schizophrenia who, after taking a cocktail of drugs containing MDMA, became convinced he had transformed into a cat. Witnesses recounted that on the day of his fall he had been prowling the local streets

---

* The transformations in Angela Carter's modern fairy tales are similarly striking.

examining the contents of bins before scaling the elm to hiss at passers-by. The police were called; he climbed higher. A dog-walker approached to watch; Gary recoiled and screeched, demonstrating a previously unexpressed terror of dogs. The police were debating how to get him down when he slipped and fell, breaking his wrist on impact. He knocked his head too and lay mewling on the grass, concussed enough to be transferred without incident to the emergency department.

The following morning Gary woke on an orthopaedic ward with a plaster cast on his arm, reluctant to discuss his experience with the hospital psychiatrist. He was discharged back to his supported accommodation – a complex of small apartments with a warden on hand to help. On visits to see how he was getting on I'd spot opened cat-food tins in his kitchen, and wonder if he was eating them. From time to time I'd ask him about that night, but he changed the subject. The last I heard, he'd adopted a couple of street cats as pets, and had cat flaps cut in the apartment door.

Early European and Near Eastern myths are full of animal transformations; some scholars take them as evidence of ancient animal worship. A glance at internet traffic suggests that the veneration of cats and dogs remains as powerful a motivation in human affairs as it ever did. Folklore traditions are full of animal transformations too, from the selkie tales of the Celtic lands, in which humans shape-shift into seals, to the spirit animal transformations of shamanism. Something these stories hold in common is that it's dangerous to lose one's hold on the human world: the selkie who spends too long as a seal forfeits their human life; the shaman who is mentally weak, or insufficiently trained, might get stuck in his or her animal skin.

'THEY ARE ALL BEASTS of burden in a sense,' wrote Thoreau, 'made to carry some portion of our thoughts.' Visit any toy shop, or watch a few television programmes made for children, and you'll see just how much humanised animals remain part of western culture. From Peter Rabbit to Stuart Little, tiger costumes to face-painting parties, adopting the skin and habits of animals offers children a liberating means of becoming fiercer, or smaller, or faster, or more agile, than they really are. For some adults, the psychosis of therianthropy may offer a comparable escape, a release from the limitations and pressures of human life.

In the late 1980s a group of psychiatrists in Massachusetts published a paper in which they described a series of twelve cases they'd seen over fourteen years at a clinic in suburban Boston. Two had suffered true lycanthropy and become wolves, two had become cats, two had become dogs, and two were 'unspecified' (their behaviour was 'crawling, howling, hooting, clawing, stamping, defaecating', and 'crawling, growling, barking'.) Of the remaining four, one had transformed into a tiger, one a rabbit, one a bird, and one – a lifetime keeper of gerbils – became his favourite pet.

There was no predominance of schizophrenia among the patients – eight were categorised as 'bipolar', two 'schizophrenic', one had a diagnosis of depression and one was described as having a 'borderline personality'. 'The presence of lycanthropy had no apparent relation to prognosis,' the authors noted: 'the delusion of being transformed into an animal may bode no more ill than any other delusion.' The most persistent transformation of all was of a young man, age twenty-four, who following a period of alcohol abuse became convinced, like Gary Hobbes, that he was a cat trapped inside a man's body. At the time the series was published this man had lived in his feline persona uninterruptedly for thirteen years.

'The patient stated that he had known that he was a cat since this secret was imparted to him by the family cat, who subsequently taught him "cat language"', the psychiatrists wrote. He held down a normal job, all the while 'he lived with cats, had sexual activity with them, hunted with them, and frequented cat night spots in preference to their human equivalent.' The psychiatrists had little hope for improvement – his belief had persisted despite various trials of antidepressants, anticonvulsants, antipsychotics and six years of psychotherapy. 'His greatest – but unrequited – love was for a tigress in the local zoo,' they concluded. 'He hoped one day to release her.'

3

Conception: The First and Second Reason for Existing

May he be ashamed who thinks badly of it.

Sir Gawain and the Green Knight

THROUGH TERM-TIME at medical school I had a job in a bar; through the summers I worked preparing dissections of human cadavers. The bar job was an education in life, and the anatomy job, I imagined at first, would be an education in death. I didn't find it macabre, but enlightening – it earned me a strong stomach and a thorough knowledge of anatomy. But it taught me nothing of death.

Only after I'd qualified as a doctor did I begin performing medicine's most doleful tasks: breaking news of terminal illness, or the death of someone loved. And working regularly on hospital wards I began to be routinely present at moments of dying: standing solemnly as someone's last breath rattled, or noticing the cooling of the skin after an unsuccessful resuscitation. It seemed somehow strange that no material change occurred at that moment of transition: the dead body was composed of the same elements as the living one of moments before. The dynamism from which life is woven, moment to moment, had merely been stilled.

It was once believed that on death the soul escaped from

an open mouth. 'Your existence is attached by a thread,' wrote Montaigne, 'it rests only on the tip of your lips.' That thread is sometimes robust and well-fastened, at others weak and loosely held. For Montaigne, death was the snapping of the thread from life's loom, the beginning of a new process of unravelling. As its converse, conception was simply the tying on of a new thread, initiating a new weave in the tapestry of life.

LEONARDO DA VINCI wrote that his earliest memory was of a red kite, a kind of hawk that feeds on carrion, swooping down to his cradle and opening his lips with its tail. Kites are masters of aerobatics – their tail shape influenced the design of Roman ships – and Leonardo watched them carefully when designing his own flying machines. Interpretations of the cradle memory vary: some see in it the ignition of his creative genius, others his perception of his exceptionality, yet others relate it tangentially to his homosexuality.

Around 1503 he painted the adult Virgin Mary seated on the lap of her mother, St Anne. Mary reaches out as if to pull Jesus back into the family, but he eludes her grasp, straddling the lamb that by convention symbolises the sacrificial crucifixion that awaits him.

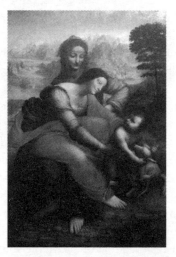

In Leonardo's day the belief that Mary had become pregnant without sex was long-established, and the notion was gathering adherents that her own conception was the same. The pope at the time brought the belief into orthodoxy. For the couple of centuries prior, Anne had been central to a medieval cult of fertility – earlier paintings show her with three daughters, each called Mary, by three husbands. At a time when women were often pregnant twenty or more times in the course of their lives, Anne's several pregnancies made her a popular saint.

Even for those who weren't saints, the creation of new life was held a divine miracle beyond the reach of human understanding. It was obvious that sex had something to do with it, but the mechanism remained a mystery. Leonardo, though, was committed to understanding every stage of human life, all the way back to its initiation. In one of his most famous cartoons, made a decade before the painting of St Anne, he attempted an X-ray anatomy of the male and female laps at the very moment of conception:

There were few precedents, and though he was a keen anatomist and dissector, most of the sexual anatomy in the cartoon was made up. His vision of the body was one in which bodily fluids are changed one into another by heat and activity. The womb he drew has a tube connecting it directly with the breasts (he thought that breast milk was transformed menstrual blood), and the womb receives a conduit of a female seminal fluid directly from the spine. His understanding of male sexual anatomy was similarly unconventional – he drew a duct from the heart into the fluid bathing the spinal cord, and other ducts bringing semen from the brain to the spine and directly into the penis. Testicles appear as little more than counterweights, holding the ducts into position. He must have had a sense of humour: over his cartoon of conception he wrote: 'I expose to men the origin of their first, and perhaps second, reason for existing.'

Twenty years after da Vinci's painting of St Anne, a German physician called Euchar Roesslin was influenced by Genesis 3:16: 'I will greatly multiply your sorrow and your conception; In pain you shall bring forth children; Your desire *shall be* for your husband, And he shall rule over you.' He suggested that the 'singular natural delight between men and women' was partial compensation for the pain of childbirth, and for both sexes, a salve against the inevitability of death.

By the 1700s, the German physician Albrecht von Haller knew that human eggs came from ovaries, but thought that sex caused each fallopian tube to stiffen and, 'surrounding and compressing the ovarium in fervent congress, [it] presses out and swallows a mature ovum.' It took seventy years before another German, Karl Ernst von Baer, actually identified a mammalian ovum (in a dog), and it wasn't until the 1930s that a human ovum was seen within a woman's fallopian tube, and modern understanding of conception began.

MUCH OF MY WORK concerns fertility and infertility: conception, contraception and, sometimes, abortion. Women come seeking assistance in losing a pregnancy or encouraging one; provoking ovulation, or preventing it. I give advice, prescribe drugs, draw inexpert cartoons of male and female anatomy. But, even today, many aspects of fertility and its rhythms remain obscure.

The creation of new life usually passes unnoticed: some women have a fleeting pain when they ovulate, but embryos can be conceived as much as twenty-four hours after that, and neither conception itself nor implantation in the womb occasions any sensation at all. It may take weeks for someone's suspicion of pregnancy to grow into a conviction, to become strong enough to go out and buy a pregnancy test.

As consultations go, it can be joyful or sombre: a woman comes into my office, sits down by the desk, and says 'I'm pregnant'. The way the words are delivered can be enough to gauge whether it's cause for celebration or dread. I take a guess which, then reply slowly with '... and how do you feel about that?' – just to be sure. 'Delighted!' I sometimes hear, or 'Awful!' Sometimes a bag opens, and urgently purchased test sticks are laid out on the desk, all showing the same blue cross or double pink line. We scrutinise them, twisting their angle to the light to make sure we're not mistaken, then repeat the test with one from my own cupboard. As the urine seeps along the reagent strip we gaze down, faces anxious and downcast, or lit with excited anticipation.

Today's tests are so sensitive that many women know within a few days of conception, when the embryo is still a thread-thin streak of cells on a disc of jelly – a streak that will define the axis of the spinal cord. When the mood in the room is excited anticipation, those moments are a treat, whether it's a longed-for baby or a welcome surprise. In those other consultations, when the mood is downcast, my questions become a little more urgent: when was your last period; how regular are they normally; when could you have conceived; have you ever been pregnant before? We're accustomed now to being in charge of our own bodies, but pregnancy is a primitive reminder that its changes are often beyond control; that bodies have their own rhythms, waypoints and fixed destinations. For some it's that inexorable quality of pregnancy that's its most terrifying aspect: a process often alienating in its otherness has been set in motion, and for the woman, whether the pregnancy proceeds or not, nothing will ever be the same again.

In most parts of the United Kingdom a woman can request the termination of a pregnancy if she feels, and two medical practitioners sign a document to agree, that there's a risk to her physical or mental health were the pregnancy to continue. The referral process is swift and discreet – I've referred happily married women whose husbands are not the father of the pregnancy, and teenagers whose lives would be misery if their parents found out. There's less of this now than there used to be: thanks to sex education and the provision of contraception, teen pregnancy rates in the UK have halved in twenty years.

I watched an IVF conception once: semen was dripped from a pipette onto a woman's eggs, layered out in a glass dish, where they fertilised almost immediately. The eggs were left multiplying in their vitrine, the multiplying cells becoming smaller and smaller as each split, until the proto-embryo was a hollow ball still comparable in size to the original egg. The development of new life doesn't bring accumulation of size or weight at first – chemical elements already present within the egg and sperm are simply woven into a new pattern. Watching a human fertilisation was both impressive and unimpressive, like watching a bee pollinating a flower.

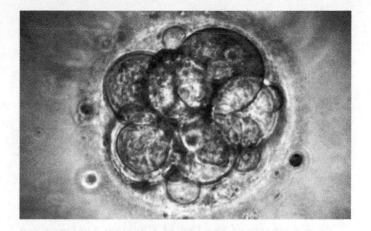

A century ago, a Massachusetts physician, Duncan MacDougall, weighed his patients immediately before and after death: the loss of mass, hence the weight of the soul, he calculated as 21 grammes. His instruments were faulty: neither the transition to death nor the conception of life occasions any change in weight, no loss or gain of mass. It is simply the cessation or initiation of all that sustain us, the commencement of a new process of transformation.

HANNAH MOLLIER was twenty-four when I met her. Her long hair was worn tied up in a knot, and between consultations it changed colour like traffic lights; she dressed in ankle-length purple or blue dresses. She and her husband Henry had moved to Scotland from the Welsh valleys, and her accent was so strong that I'd often ask her to repeat herself. One day in clinic she opened her bag and three pregnancy tests tumbled out onto my desk. 'I'm pregnant,' she said.

'And how do you feel about that?' I asked her.

'It wasn't planned if that's what you mean, but I'm going through with it.' We talked about vitamins and midwives, ultrasound scans and morning sickness, and I referred her to the antenatal clinic.

I saw her regularly through the pregnancy, which was dreadful for her: high blood pressure, nausea, heartburn, and back pain so severe she could hardly walk. 'There'll be no more after this one,' she told me in her lilting, sing-song accent. 'One is enough.'

Six weeks following the delivery she brought the baby to see me – a delicate little girl with dark eyes like ink spots and a pelage of translucent, downy fur. After I'd completed the screening checks on her daughter, and examined the scar of her caesarean section for how well it had healed, we discussed the options for contraception: she left with a prescription for contraceptive pills. 'They've a failure rate of about 1 per cent,' I told her: 'it's important to take them at around the same time every day.'

Three months later she was back in clinic, pushing a pram ahead of her. When I went to call her from the waiting room, I noticed she was sitting beside another patient of mine who was just embarking on her third cycle of IVF.

'I'm pregnant again!' Hannah said, as she negotiated the pram through the office doorway. She sat down, and with one arm continued to rock the pram.

'And how do you feel about that?' I asked.

'It's a nightmare, isn't it? I've not recovered from the last time. I knew right away: feeling sick, sore breasts ...' She paused a moment, her expression shifting as she realised why I'd asked. 'But we're going through with it, Henry and me – our minds are made up.'

Hannah's second pregnancy was more gruelling for her than the first – we met every two to three weeks, juggling medications for sickness, for heartburn, for back pain and worsening sciatica. Towards the end she became incontinent of urine, struggled to leave her flat, and could barely sleep. The platelet count in her blood dropped, her blood pressure rose, and the gynaecologists offered to deliver the baby by caesarean section again. 'I'm definitely not having any more,' she told me, limping around her flat when

I called in to see her. 'Can't they just tie my tubes while they're in there?'

'I'll ask,' I said, and wrote a letter to the department of obstetrics and gynaecology.

Two weeks later a message arrived: 'Female sterilisation in a woman as young as Hannah is inadvisable,' she'd replied. 'Rates of regret are high. We will offer a contraceptive implant at the time of discharge from hospital.'

IT TOOK UNTIL the nineteenth century for medicine to catch up with da Vinci's research, when a series of mostly German gynaecologists pondered the anatomy of conception. They scrutinised physical changes during intercourse, and guessed their effects on the likelihood of conception. They queried which sexual positions had the best chance of success, and whether sex during pregnancy was dangerous. They theorised with one another about whether the womb itself altered its shape or position during orgasm. None of them were women.

In 1933, just as physiologists were beginning to understand human fertility and the timing of ovulation, pornography laws in the United States relaxed enough for a New Jersey physician called Robert Dickinson to publish his own research. Dickinson believed that anatomical science needed to get away from the dead bodies in the dissection room, and occupy itself instead with living human beings. As a gynaecologist he was challenged daily to figure out why some couples struggled to conceive, and realised that society's reluctance to discuss sex freely was the cause not just of enormous misery, but even of infertility. 'Perhaps,' he wrote, 'this shyness is begotten by the certainty that such study cannot be freed from the warp of personal experience, the bias of individual prejudice, and, above all, from the implication of prurience.' He begins a chapter called 'Anatomy of Coitus' with an observation of the centrality of sex in the perpetuation of human life: 'No bodily function of human beings may challenge sex intercourse for far reaching effects from a single act, or for manifold implications based on short total time of action. In the single act new life or no life can hang on seconds.'

It was 'no life' that most concerned him – whether conception was hoped for, or whether it was to be prevented – and his book includes a chapter on contraceptive devices, and on methods of abortion. One passage describes how to carry out a simultaneous abortion and sterilisation. Carrying out the two procedures through a single abdominal opening gave women a single scar, and for the many who approached him in secret, he argued it offered 'a better alibi'. One of his illustrations attempts to delineate, in profile, like Leonardo, the most important journey any of us ever made, when our mother's ovum and our father's sperm came together.

Dickinson's final section is on the anatomy of different sexual positions, and in particular how they affect the pooling of semen at the cervix, and the likelihood of conception. He thought that a varied sex life would help conception, but that wasn't his only concern:

> Artistry avoids monotony. This applies not alone to variety in action but to variety in atmosphere and adventure, to the notion of sea and sky as none too spacious and spring woods or moonlight none too gracious as background and as setting for rapture and splendour.

Following Dickinson, more precise representations of the anatomy of conception weren't possible until the 1990s, when accurate MRI scanners became available. A Dutch physiologist, radiologist, anthropologist and gynaecologist solicited the help of seven couples who agreed to have sex inside an MRI scanner (the anthropologist and her partner also volunteered). Their paper begins by acknowledging how little was known about the anatomy of sex, and commenting that even six decades after Dickinson, research was still being held back by the fear of being seen as prurient. They demonstrated changes in the position of the womb during female arousal, and noticed that Dickinson had been wrong about the shape of the penis during intercourse. They demonstrated striking changes in the blood supply to the vagina during sex.

Only one of the couples involved, the anthropologist and her partner, managed to sustain intercourse long enough for the scanner to take accurate images. 'The reason might be that they were the only participants in the real sense,' the paper concludes, 'involved in the research right from the beginning ... and as amateur street acrobats they are trained and were used to performing under stress.'

WHEN I SAW HANNAH after her second delivery she was pushing a double pram. I asked how she was coping with two babies – her daughter was just fourteen months old – and she gave a hollow laugh. 'We can cope,' she said; 'he's good, my Henry – together we manage.' Her second daughter was more unsettled than her first had been; nights were disrupted, and both she and Henry were exhausted. But they were still able to laugh. Just. She was keen to show me the site of her contraceptive implant. It was high on the inside of her left arm, just under the skin – about the size and thickness of a matchstick, but smooth and flexible. 'I don't know why I need to bother with contraception,' she said and gave a ribald laugh. 'Sex is the last thing on either of our minds.'

When the youngest was about four months old I came to work to find a note on my desk: 'Call Hannah Mollier,' it said, 'it's urgent.'

'You're never going to believe this, Dr Francis,' she said down the telephone. 'I'm pregnant again.'

'... and how do you feel about—'

'I can't go through with this, I just can't, I don't think my body can take it.' The line went quiet for a few seconds. 'I hate the idea of an abortion, but I'm going to have to. I could hardly even walk the last time, couldn't sleep, was peeing myself. I think I need an abortion. Don't you think I need one, on medical grounds?'

She was early in the pregnancy, and could only have conceived a few days previously. I phoned the obstetrics and gynaecology department explaining her situation, her two young babies, her disabling back pain worsened by pregnancy, the failure of contraception. Abortion clinics send their appointments to the referring clinic rather than to a home address (too many women still have to seek abortions in secret), and so the following day I rang Hannah with the place and time for her to attend for what's called an 'early medical' abortion. She met a counsellor who explored her choices, and explained how she'd be given a tablet to block hormones of pregnancy then, a day later, a pessary to put inside the vagina to encourage the shedding of womb lining.

We spoke on the phone the following week. 'You'll never guess,' she told me. 'It didn't work. I'm still pregnant. They say it's a one in a thousand chance.'

Again she met the counsellors, again she took the tablet; again she was given a pessary to take home, and again it didn't work.

'By my calculations that makes me one in a million,' she said. I wondered if the pessary had failed, or whether once home, Hannah had felt unable to use it.

I saw Hannah the following week, back in clinic to have the contraceptive implant taken out of her arm. The counsellors had offered her a decisive surgical termination, but she'd turned them down. 'I've decided to go ahead with it,' she told me, shuffling her double pram forwards and backwards as she spoke. 'Why didn't those tablets work?' she asked.

'No idea,' I said, shaking my head. 'I guess you're right – you must be one in a million.'

'Well, if this baby wants to stay so much, maybe I should let it.' The lilt of her accent rose up and down, lifting and dropping like a needle on a running stitch.

4

Sleep: The Chamber of Dreams

I had never heard mention before then of any gods that could make
people sleep, nor to wake.

Chaucer, *The Book of the Duchess*

SOME PATIENTS ATTEND my clinic complaining of flitting
symptoms that veer from one part of the body to another.
As soon as I begin to get an understanding of one symptom
(knee pain, say, or stomach cramps) the narrative shifts, and
I'm asked to come to terms with another. It's as if each
symptom recounted is of less importance than the suffering I'm being asked to acknowledge. To recast the focus of
the conversation into the sufferer's mental and emotional
life, drawing it away from the repetitive listing of ever more
physical symptoms, it can be enough to ask: 'How is your
sleep?'

'Terrible,' I'm sometimes told, or 'Too good – I'm never
out of bed.' Chronic pain can cause agitated and unrefreshing sleep, but so can a restless, agitated mind. Oversleeping
can mean thyroid deficiency, but it can also suggest being in
retreat from the world. For many people, being asked about
sleep isn't as threatening as being asked about anxieties or
despondencies.

Many of the serial insomniacs I meet can't switch off

their attention – every time they glide towards sleep some controlling, rational part of their mind jerks them awake. Brain scans show that when sleeping the analytical parts of our brains tend to fall silent, while more instinctual, emotional areas come alive. To fall asleep is a kind of abandonment, of consciousness as well as of the body; sleep's inherent lack of control can make it a terrifying prospect for some. Often there's an urgency just to get some sleep: the pills to achieve this can be dangerously addictive but, for the most part, effective. Sedatives like valerian are among the oldest known drugs, and opium too has been used for millennia.

It's estimated that about 10 per cent of the world's population suffer chronic insomnia – a 'symptom' experienced by the patient, not a 'diagnosis' implying a particular medical cause – and the proportion who sleep poorly is higher still. No one can say exactly why we have to sleep, but every organism goes through alternating periods of repose and activity. Some cetaceans, seals, and birds even sleep with one half of their brains at a time, suggesting that the process is so important that it must not be suspended for long: vital cerebral hygiene is at stake. Neural processes engaged through sleep are thought to remove waste material produced by brain cells, restore aspects of the body's function, and repair injured tissues. Children sleep more than adults because their brains are constantly learning, and because they have to grow so much – it's during sleep that growth hormone is generated by the body. The longer we're awake the more a chemical called adenosine accumulates in our neural tissues. Vital for cellular energy metabolism, too much adenosine makes us feel terrible, but sleep returns its levels to normal.*

---

* We need sleep to live: there is a genetic condition called 'Familial Fatal Insomnia' in which a progressive intractable insomnia, in step with a deteriorating dementia, leads to death. It is thankfully extremely rare.

Different phases of sleep seem to perform different functions: REM sleep, in which the majority of dreaming occurs, is important for memory consolidation (or perhaps the systematic forgetting of useless information*), while without 'slow wave' sleep we may wake feeling unrefreshed. (REM means 'rapid eye movement'; though the body is paralysed, the muscles around the eyes continue to move.) We experience REM every ninety minutes or so while we sleep – most adults have four or five episodes of it each night. Phases of 'non-REM' sleep have traditionally been divided into four stages, I–IV, but this classification has been challenged as overly simplistic.

Much about the detail and the mechanisms of sleep remains mysterious. Newborn babies spend about half their sleep time in REM, and adults about a quarter. The deepest phases of sleep, when the brain's EEG tracings show deep coordinated pulses in neural activity, also diminish as we age – some elderly people don't enter the deepest phase of slow wave sleep at all. REM is triggered by a tiny bunch of neurons that spring from deep in the brainstem and flow into a region at the core of the brain called the thalamus. When they activate, REM is enabled. Only mammals and birds have REM. If you wake someone during REM, 90 per cent of the time they'll report having a dream.

From the 1950s to the 1990s it was largely assumed that to be in REM sleep *was* to be in a dream, but more recently that's been shown to be wrong. If you wake someone during non-REM sleep, there's still a 10 per cent chance they'll report a dream, though those dreams are usually more conceptual and less vivid than dreams reported during REM.

Sleep might be relatively straightforward to grant with drugs, but recurrent, distressing dreams are a more difficult problem. But listening to the narrative within dreams, and

---

*Francis Crick, one of the discoverers of DNA's structure, believed that this was the purpose of REM sleep.

exploring their associations, can offer a welcome space in which to explore unarticulated anxieties and preoccupations. I'm not a psychoanalyst, but listening to the content of my patients' dreams can often be helpful in exploring the challenges and complexities of their lives. Here are some recurrent dreams I have heard in the consulting room, only in the past year:

An elderly man finds himself running through a labyrinth of corridors, opening and closing the silvered doors of rooms. Sometimes he enters a room, and pulls out all the drawers – he's looking for something, but doesn't know what. A list in his pocket urges him on, a list he's sure is incomplete. As the dream progresses he grows more frantic until he wakes with a start, eyes wet with tears, his heart pounding against his ribs.

A successful museum curator with a high public profile and onerous administrative responsibilities dreams herself as a surgeon, standing over a slit body. Nurses surround her in silent expectation; there are entrails hanging out, and she can't figure out how to put them back in.

A young man, violated and abused by his parents as a child, is haunted by persistent recurrent dreams of cartoon characters. Sometimes they fly around his head, taunting and mocking him. Sometimes they humiliate him, or one another. He wakes from these dreams electrified by horror, and fears sleep.

THERE'S A DREAMLIKE QUALITY to Ovid's *Metamorphoses*; the reader is aware of being drawn into a strange, hallucinatory space. In Book XI the dream-god Morpheus is described as living at the bounds of the earth, in a cave surrounded by opium poppies. The waters of the river Lethe, which springs from the cave, 'invite slumber as they glide'; dark, soporific mists emanate from the earth. Morpheus's father Somnus, the god of sleep, lies dozing on a vast ebony couch in the cave. He's surrounded by the insubstantial forms of numberless dreams, 'as many as the harvest bears ears of corn, the wood green leaves, or as the sands cast up on the shore'.

Morpheus means 'shape-maker' – he can take any human shape. His purpose is to act out the dreams of mortals, in order to send them portents. That dreams are charged with divine significance was taken for granted among the Near Eastern and Mediterranean cultures which nourished Ovid's thought: the Babylonian *Epic of Gilgamesh* has both the eponymous hero and his alter ego Enkidu receiving clairvoyant dreams. The power of dreaming is celebrated in the Hebrew scriptures with the story of Joseph, a young Hebrew from Canaan who's supremely adept at the interpretation of God-given dreams. There are numerous other episodes in Egyptian, Mesopotamian and Greek culture that testify to the importance of understanding the messages within dreams.

One of the founding texts of psychoanalysis is Freud's *The Interpretation of Dreams* – a title he took from a two-thousand-year-old work by an Ionian Greek called Artemidorus ('*Oneirocritica*'). Freud didn't believe that dreams come from the gods, but neither did he see them as the flotsam of a chaotic, ungoverned mind – he saw them as the guardians of sleep. Our restless minds would wake us ceaselessly, Freud said, if it weren't for the transformative power of dreaming. Just as Morpheus changed shape in order to act out our dreams, so dreaming transforms our fear, shame and dark ambitions into the narratives of our dreams. For Ovid, the dream-god Morpheus comes as a storyteller, and his fictions illuminate deeper truths.

'THALAMUS' MEANS 'inner chamber'. The thalamus lies beneath the mushroom folds of the cerebral cortex, under the caves of the cerebral ventricles. I've examined them at autopsy: twinned packets of grey matter the colour and consistency of alluvial clay. Their function is to pass on sensory information towards the cerebral cortex, filtering and relaying all that we see, hear and touch. The world flows to us through the networks and synapses of the thalamus, and when sedative drugs make us sleep, it's in part because those drugs change thalamic function.

Each of the senses is apportioned a thalamic 'nucleus', and within each nucleus millions of connections are humming and clicking in communication with one another and with the cortex. Sight passes through to the back of the brain, where it's perceived a couple of inches above the bones of the neck. Hearing rises up and out in a radiation to be processed beneath the ears themselves.* Touch is perceived in a ribbon of cortex wrapped like a headphone band across the top of the brain. Smell and taste – our earthiest, most primitive senses – are different: they pass directly into the brain's underbelly, where they mingle with the emotional centres involved in hunger and lust, fear and memory. The cortex that makes sense of smell and taste is more primitive too – structured in just four layers instead of six – a hangover from our reptilian evolutionary past. It's the primitive way in which smell and taste are perceived that makes them so evocative of our past, and so intimately associated with feelings like nostalgia or disgust.

The brain's world is electrical: it's through electricity that nerve cells communicate with one another, and it is through manipulating each cell's electrical voltage that thalamic neurons block or transmit sense information. Each thalamic neuron answers to the rhythm of the sense that it serves. The activity of its neurons can be imagined as a million desynchronised drum machines, pounding out a million different rhythms, each one responding to a different sense-impression. In addition to the classical five senses, ceaseless torrents of data inform the cortex

---

* A paradox being that the noises heard in the right ear are processed in the cortex beneath the left, and vice versa.

moment to moment of our balance, motion, temperature, thirst, hunger, the tension and position of every muscle and tendon of the body, the fullness or emptiness of our bladder and rectum, and the pressure of air in the lungs and windpipe, not to mention all the higher-order reflections, perceptions and memories that clatter constantly through our waking minds. The din of all this would deafen us if we weren't so skilled at directing our attention to just two or three sensations at a time. But when it comes to sleeping, even a few of the millions of sensations pressing in on us would be distracting. To permit the brain to rest it's not enough just to direct our attention, we have to slam the gate of the senses shut.

When we begin to drift towards sleep, one among many changes is that ions of potassium leach out through the wetsuit-tight membranes that clothe each thalamic cell, and into the surrounding extracellular fluid. The leaching occurs because of the change in shape of a tiny membrane channel called 'K_{2P}': twin pores open within the channel's structure and positively charged potassium ions glide out. The electrical charge of the neuron drops with the departure of the potassium, and the speed of thalamic neurons' firing slows as a consequence. Awake, millions of syncopated rhythms convey all the complexity of the world around us. Asleep, those neurons slow to a deep, harmonised beat that shields us from awareness. When we shake ourselves awake the reverse occurs: K_{2P} channels narrow and close, the voltage in the thalamic neurons rises, and each begins again to faithfully transmit information to the cerebral hemispheres about the outside world.

K_{2P} channels aren't unique to humans – they were first identified in pond snails. They're not unique to the brain either – you can find them in the kidney and in the pancreas (where their function is less thoroughly understood). We know they're involved in sleep because when scientists deliver anaesthetic gases or sedative drugs to pond snails, their K_{2P} channels open, and the snails become sluggish. Even pond snails sleep. Maybe they even dream.

Artemidorus, the Greek author of *Oneirocritica*, didn't get caught up in the question of whether dreams come from the gods or from the self – he said only that when we experience recurring dreams, 'our spirit admonishes and foretells us affectionately the self-same thing worthy to be thought upon.' I appreciate the gentleness of that 'affectionately'; some of my own consultations become quiet, mutual reflections on what recurring dreams might mean. The sites where dreaming takes place within the brain are poorly understood, and they can be a dangerous territory – a realm of primitive emotion we explore at our peril. Drugs like amphetamines tap into the same areas of the brain as dreaming when they gift energy and elation; if those same regions become ungoverned, the waking nightmare of psychosis may break through. In clinic, I ask about dreams cautiously, aware not just that they're deeply private, but that their content carries power.

I began to ask those of my patients who experience recurrent nightmares what their spirit could be 'affectionately admonishing' them to contemplate. I asked dreamer one, who found himself nightly running through corridors opening and closing doors, to talk more to me about his personal history. His wife and both his children had died in appalling circumstances many years before (car crash, cancer, suicide). If there was any eloquence to his dream, it perhaps expressed anguish over all that had been left unsaid between himself, his wife, and his children. There was a horror that came from his knowledge that he could never substitute his life for theirs. Exploring this as a potential meaning didn't diminish the frequency of his dreams, but it did allow him to articulate something of the depth of his grief. The intimacy that grew between us through those discussions made it easier, I hope, to discuss other fears and anxieties. I couldn't cure him of grief, but through discussions of his dreams we created a space for that grief to be voiced.

Dreamer two had dreamed herself a surgeon uncertain how to proceed; when she began to talk about that terror she moved naturally, and without being prompted, into a disclosure of her childhood, her career choices, and her parent's high ambitions for her – they always put on pressure to transcend the family's modest background. She admitted that she never expected to be promoted so highly, and often worried that those around her thought her not up to the responsibilities of her job. When we were able to discuss those feelings of inadequacy – of being an imposter in her role – she went on to list all the reasons she was, in truth, ideally qualified for her post.

For dreamer three, who repeatedly experienced taunting and tormenting at the hands of cartoon characters, the physical and emotional betrayals he suffered as a small child were too raw to begin approaching with words: he found himself unable to talk about them. We decided instead to suppress the dreams with drugs. There's a drug called clonazepam that blunts and attenuates our dreams, or at least subdues the memory of them. I began a regular prescription of clonazepam for him, to be taken until such time as he feels able to talk about the tragic abuse of his past, either with me or with a counsellor – a time we acknowledged might never come.

5

Bodybuilding: Unhelmed by Fury

If you want to be strong, you must accustom your body to be the servant of your mind, and train it with toil and sweat.

Prodicus, *On Hercules*

ONE OF THE FIRST CONSTELLATIONS I learned to recognise was that of Hercules: a box of stars radiating flailing, half-bent limbs. Look for the Pole Star, then follow the tiny saucepan handle of Ursa Minor, and you're not far off. As a child, I had a pop-up book about astronomy, and over starry bones it showed a greyed-out Hercules kneeling, club in hand, about to deal a death blow to the serpent Draco.

I knew the story of Hercules because my schoolteacher had organised a project on Greek mythology. According to the myth, Draco was a snake-like creature guarding an apple tree in a sacred garden when Hercules (or, as the Greeks named him, Heracles) clubbed him to death. I don't remember her pointing out the parallels with the story of the Garden of Eden, but I do remember her asking us to make drawings of Hercules's twelve labours. I sketched mountains of shit in the Augean stables, and puddles of blood under the Nemean lion (his 'thirteenth' labour, the impregnation of fifty virgins in a single night, was never mentioned). He was so strong, the teacher said, that when a superhuman being called Atlas tired of holding up the heavens, Hercules was the only mortal powerful enough to take on the task.

In the most usual telling of the myth Hercules was the son of Zeus, result of one of his many illegitimate affairs. Zeus's wife Hera tried to prevent the birth, directing magic spells at Hercules's mother while clamping her own thighs tightly together. This was an integral part of the spell, and Hera was tricked into uncrossing her legs; the enchantment broke, and Hercules survived his first labour. It was immediately apparent that the boy was strong: in his cot he strangled the snakes that Hera sent to kill him, and the prophet Tiresias augured that he would accomplish great deeds.

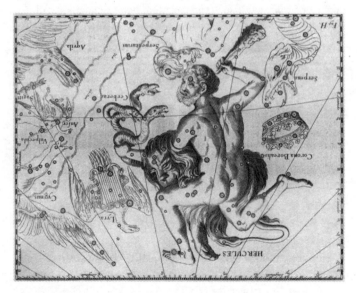

HARRY ALKMAN ABUSED anabolic steroids. It wasn't his muscles that gave me the clue, but his skin: no matter what treatment I gave, his acne remained disastrous. I tried everything in the armoury: lotions and astringents, antibiotics and vitamin A, but his shoulders, neck and cheeks continued to erupt with pustules which scarred to pits, as if raindrops had fallen on the dust of his skin. I was new to medicine when we met, with an innocent belief in my patients' honesty. While discussing Harry's acne at a coffee break one day, a more experienced colleague suggested: 'Ask again what else he's taking.'

At our next appointment I asked Harry if he was *sure* he never took anything I hadn't prescribed; he confessed he'd been buying steroids online for the last four years. 'Which one?' I asked.

'One?' he said, surprised by my ignorance. 'No one takes just one.'

'Well, what *do* you take?'

'Well, I started with testosterone and some Dianabol. That's to bulk you up, for the first twelve weeks. And also anastrozole to stop man-boobs.' I knew anastrozole as a hormonal treatment for women with breast cancer.

'And then?'

'Well, that depends on what you want to achieve. To get more definition you'd usually switch the type of testosterone, and add in something like Anavar. But keep going with the anastrozole.'

'So you said that's for starters. What do you take once you've moved up a level?'

'There are plenty of schedules out there,' he said, 'Masteron, Equipoise, Decanate, Nandrone, human growth hormone ...'

I interrupted: 'Your acne won't get better until you stop taking those steroids. They're making your skin oily, which brings on the spots and scarring.' I ran through some of the other risks of steroids: heart failure through its effect on cardiac muscle, diabetes, infertility, depression, uncontainable bouts of rage. He listened politely; in his lap I could see the skin over his knuckles tightening and relaxing.

'If you don't want to help me with my acne just say so,' he said finally. 'But I know what I'm doing. I've never felt better.'

THE FIRST BODYBUILDER in the modern sense was a nine-teenth-century German circus strongman called Friedrich Müller, who adopted the stage name Eugen Sandow. He claimed to have been inspired by a famous Roman statue of Hercules, the 'Farnese'. In his manifesto 'Body-Build-ing', Sandow coined a phrase as well as an industry – to emphasise the self-improvement ethos of his new sport, he subtitled it 'Man in the Making'. He patented a regime of clean living and weight training that resonated with the fin-de-siècle obsession with colonial strength and self-determination. In 1901 he conceived a public contest to find the world's best physique: it was organised at the Royal Albert Hall in London, and judged by the author and physician Arthur Conan Doyle and the sculptor and fitness enthusiast Charles Bennett Lawes. Opening the show was a troupe of gymnasts from the London Orphan Asylum. The contestants paraded on stage, dressed in black tights and animal skins, striking poses from famous statues of antiq-uity. Sandow presented the winner with a golden statue of himself holding a Herculean pose.

Sandow must have had immense willpower; he claimed he had been a weakling until he was inspired by the statue of Hercules to build up his muscles. He sold his patented techniques by mail order, and from the outset his aim was an aesthetic one: mimicry of classical statuary rather than feats of particular strength. In the journey from circus strongman to the Albert Hall he made a leap of respectability; adopting classical motifs gave the endeavour a dignity and acceptance which broadened its audience. That audience grew expo-nentially with the advent of cinema: after 1910, Italian films like *Cabiria*, *Marcantonio e Cleopatra*, and *Quo Vadis?* all led with Herculean muscle-men, and borrowed heavily from the classics. The films were phenomenally successful across Europe and the United States, and their actors became celebrities – feted for their muscles rather than their acting skills or good looks. By the 1960s, the films were epic in

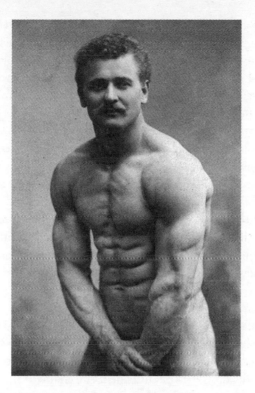

scope: Steve Reeves's *Hercules* and *Hercules Unchained* set the tone for bodybuilders as actors. Others followed: Arnold Schwarzenegger (*Hercules in New York*), Mickey Hargitay (*The Loves of Hercules*) and Ralf Moeller (*Gladiator*).

In his memoir *The Education of a Bodybuilder*, Arnold Schwarzenegger wrote of how at the age of fifteen he first visited a gym in Austria and became intoxicated by the idea of transforming his body. The men who took him on as a protégé were huge, brutal but profoundly admirable – he sought specifically to emulate their 'Herculean' looks. His account of his first summer in the gym is steeped in a kind of sexual intoxication: Schwarzenegger felt turned on by the feeling of his muscles expanding, and dreamed of growing ever more gigantic. He modelled his own training schedule on that of the bodybuilding actor Reg Park (star of *Hercules and the Conquest of Atlantis*). Park advocated a kind of sculptural bodybuilding, which involved first pumping the muscles up, and then finessing the definition of each one.* Like an autoerotic Pygmalion, Schwarzenegger fell more deeply in love with his body as he sculpted it.

On the subject of steroids, Schwarzenegger is coy: his *Encyclopedia of Modern Bodybuilding* slips a discussion of performance-enhancing drugs into the last couple of pages. Every great bodybuilder uses steroids, he declares, but they do so only as a final polish to a body already honed to near-perfection through *effort*. Steroids, he says, are essential if you want to keep your edge – an edge as much mental as physical. The drugs don't just help build muscle faster and stronger, they bring on an aggression that facilitates a ferociously competitive attitude to training.

FROM MY DESK I usually had warning that Harry Alkman was coming to clinic – his voice like a chain-gang foreman carrying from the hallway as he argued with the receptionists, or his dogs barking outside as he chained them to the surgery steps. He had three Staffordshire bull terriers – pale, muscled and belligerent.

After the conversation about his acne I didn't see him for a few months. The next time I heard those dogs barking, I went out to the waiting room to find him sitting with his girlfriend Tanya. She was silent in the corner: pale, and nervous, her ginger hair straggling over a grey tracksuit top. Harry sat with legs spread, occupying the space of three chairs. The cloth of his T-shirt bulged as if crammed with snakes.

'You've got to help him with his temper,' Tanya said tentatively, as they sat down together in my office. Her voice

---

* In 1972, after winning Mr Universe, Schwarzenegger was invited to Park's home in Johannesburg. Park criticised the definition of his calves, and instructed Schwarzenegger on how to improve them.

was like a child's whisper. 'It's getting out of hand.' Harry's skin looked better, and I asked if he was still taking steroids.

He laughed. 'Maybe I tried a new regime,' he said.

'He won't listen to what I say,' said Tanya, her eyes pressing on me.

'To be honest, he doesn't tend to listen to me either,' I said.

A few nights previously they had been having an argument and Harry had lashed out at her; she dodged, and his fist hit the wall. The impact snapped a bone. He held up the hand as evidence, bandaged in the emergency department. 'See what she made me do? You've got to give me something to calm down.'

'You're responsible for your own actions,' I said, as calmly as I could. 'And if you cut out the steroids you'll get less angry.' I reached down into the drawer for a leaflet titled 'Alternatives to Violence', circled the phone number on the front, and handed it over. The leaflet carried a portrait of a pensive young man, heavily muscled, above the legend: 'Be Who You Want To Be: Respect yourself, Listen to others, Get on with people.'

'You have to stop those steroids,' I repeated. 'And Tanya, if he threatens you or hurts you – phone the police.'

She came a week later without him, and I told her about the local women's shelter where she could go if she ever felt unsafe at home. She already had their number.

THERE'S YET ANOTHER VERSION of Hercules's myth, dramatised by the Greek playwright Euripides, in which, on the completion of his twelve labours, Hercules returns home to his wife Megara and their three sons. In this telling, Hera can't bear to see Hercules happy after his labours, so from her viewpoint on Mount Olympus she sends a furious madness upon him. Euripides describes the change: 'He was no longer himself; his eyes were rolling; he was distraught; his eyeballs were bloodshot, and foam was oozing down his bearded cheek. He spoke with a madman's laugh.' Hera's spell makes Hercules believe that Megara and his children are enemies; boiling with rage he turns on them. He slaughters one son with an arrow; his second son pleads with him but Hercules, absorbed in his frenzy, clubs the boy to death and tramples on his bones. He then turns on his wife and third son, shooting a single arrow through both bodies. Finally, his family slaughtered, he turns on his foster father Amphitryon but the goddess Pallas intervenes, hurling a rock at his breast. As it hits home his 'frenzied thirst for blood' fades; he falls to the floor and into an enchanted sleep.

MANY CULTURES HAVE STORIES of muscle-bound strongmen, unhelmed by fury. In medieval Norse culture these men were much valued in battle: they were called 'berserks', or 'bear-shirts', transformed by their bloodlust to become as much bears as men. The Germans too had a word for that altered state: 'mordlust', a lust for death. The Anglo-Saxons had Beowulf; the Irish, Cú Chulainn; in Hindu mythology, Krishna; for the Babylonians, Gilgamesh. There are resonances and echoes with the battle-trance of Achilles. The Hebrew Bible has the story of Samson, a Herculean strongman who, like his Greek counterpart, kills a lion with his bare hands, pulls down buildings and lays waste to an army (but where Hercules has his bow and arrows, Samson is armed with an ass's jawbone). Just as the Greek myth gives Hercules three earthly 'wives' in quick succession, the Hebrew story offers Samson the same.

Anabolic steroids can make an already irascible temper far worse – there are a few accounts in the medical literature of murder committed under their influence. Weight training without steroids can enhance well-being by boosting testosterone, but it can also intensify background aggression. A study conducted in a male prison showed that the most aggressive men had higher testosterone levels. Men born with doubled 'Y' chromosomes instead of the usual single

'Y' don't just have more testosterone, there is some evidence to suggest that they are over-represented in the prison population, possibly through greater propensity to short-tempered violence. Anecdotal evidence suggests that when adolescent boys are in the midst of the testosterone boost of puberty they get into more fights, and become more argumentative at home. Like the madness of Hercules, unnatural levels of testosterone can ignite furies that consume the individual, even as they threaten everyone around him.

MEN WHO TAKE ANABOLIC STEROIDS for a length of time usually become infertile, because artificial testosterone inhibits the body from making its own. Their testicles shrink, and their sperm count drops. As if in awareness of the paradoxical effects of excessive testosterone, many of the greatest strongmen in mythology pass through a phase of feminisation: Thor goes through a period dressing as a woman, as does Krishna. One of the Greek myths of Hercules tells that in one of his three marriages he stayed home to cook and clean, while his wife went out hunting and fighting. In one version of the story of the Trojan War, Achilles's mother tries to keep him home by dressing him as a girl (he is betrayed when the Greek army passes through the village, and he can't resist fondling their weapons).

The next time I saw Harry there was no warning – no barking of dogs, no yelling at the reception desk. He was sitting quietly in the waiting room when I went to call him, wearing a loose hooded sweatshirt. As he sat down in the chair of my office, he placed a piece of paper on the desk.

'What's this?' I asked.

'My new regime. I've come to see what you think.'

The piece of paper had a list of medications on it, and none of them were anabolic steroids.

'So have you stopped taking testosterone?' I asked him.

'Yep – I've brought it down slowly. Tanya and I are going to have kids. I've come to see if you'll help.'

'Well, I can't prescribe any of this stuff for you – most of these are IVF drugs for women. They're not licensed for use in men.'

'I don't need you to prescribe them for me – I'll get them and inject them myself. I just wanted to know what you think of the regime, and if you'll send the sperm count test afterwards, to see if it's worked.'

Harry had it all worked out: his research had told him to arrange a week of daily injections with a hormone to stimulate his testicles. Then he'd start a drug which in women leads to hyperovulation, but in men can kick-start the production of sperm. Anastrozole was on the regime again – this time to prevent Harry's natural testosterone being converted into oestrogen by the body.* The sperm he produced would at first be very sluggish, so after a month he'd take a fairly low dose of another drug to promote agility and mobility of the new sperm.

I phoned a colleague who specialises in endocrinology – the study of hormones – to ask him about the regime. 'Will it work?' I asked him.

'Sadly, it probably will,' he said. 'But most bodybuilders do this every so often, just to make sure their testes are still working. As soon as they get the reassurance of a normal sperm count, they go back on the steroids.'

BODYBUILDING COULD BE DESCRIBED as a species of addiction, both to the mental rush when blood surges to the brain fresh from swollen muscles, known as 'pump', and to a body shape perceived to be superior. A couple of decades ago it was thought of as a modern neurosis – a 'body dysmorphic disorder' responding to a contemporary

---

* Men who have one testicle removed often experience a flare of testosterone production from the remaining one. It swells in size, and breast tissue beneath their nipples may swell as the newly released testosterone is converted to oestrogen.

crisis in masculinity. For some bodybuilders there may be a fragment of truth in that, but Eugen Sandow and Arnold Schwarzenegger are emblematic of a dream that has been around for as long as humans have admired strength.

In most of the Greek myths of Hercules he is born strong, but in a story recorded by Xenophon, one of Plato's pupils, there was a moment in the hero's adolescence when he had to make a choice between a life of strength or a life of ease. Walking along a path one day, Hercules encounters two women who present him with a decision. He could choose a path of comfort through life or a path of difficulty. The path of difficulty would require great effort but would result in a commensurate measure of honour. He could be strong, but that strength wouldn't come as the free gift from a god or through taking a drug – it would come only through the exercise of will. He chose the path of difficulty: 'For of all things good and fair, the gods give nothing to man without toil and effort.'

6

Scalp: Of Horns, Terror and Glory

My hair is grey, but not with years,
Nor grew it white
In a single night,
As men's have grown from sudden fears.

Lord Byron, The Prisoner of Chillon

ON A JOURNEY THE LENGTH of the New York subway I once attempted a survey of the hairstyles of everyone who entered my carriage. There were spray-backs of radiant gold; ringlets of bouncing delight; dreadlocks and crew cuts; forelocks and permanent waves. A multiplicity of braids, plaits, ponytails, pigtails, tresses, tufts and knots. I counted Afros, mullets and tonsures. There were quiffs, coiffures, streaks of white and rainbow-dyes of colour. There were also fungal patches of ringworm and balding patches of alopecia.

Even the bald scalps showed a wealth of diversity: some were pockmarked like asteroids, others looked worn down and freckled – sandstone sculptures under acid rain. Some had swatches of bruises, others were glossy as polished mahogany. Some were wrinkled, others suave, some scratched like glacial erratics. I saw scalps that were crusted with psoriasis, others with sun damage and dermatitis. I didn't see anyone with horns.

THE SCALP HAS one of the best blood supplies in the body: wide arterial trunks ascend into it from each side of the face, and when it gets wounded, blood can spurt a couple of centimetres into the air. Scalp skin is tough, and its wounds satisfying to stitch – in the emergency department I often start with a few tight silk sutures to halt the bleeding, and then finish the job with staples or glue. 'Superglue' was invented during the Vietnam War for the express purpose of repairing briskly bleeding wounds like those of the scalp. Only the tongue and cheek heal quicker, thanks to their more generous blood supply. The scalp is among the thickest skin on the body, at around 1 mm (skin thickness varies from 0.05 mm in the eyelids and behind the ears, to 1.5 mm on the palms and soles of our feet). Women have thicker skin on their scalps than men, and bald, elderly men the thinnest scalps of all. All this variety across the acreage of the body's surface makes skin our largest and heaviest organ, oddly and unjustifiably overlooked by most medical training.

Training in every speciality involved being summoned to 'interesting cases' and then adding them to an inner register of experience, but being a medical student in Dermatology felt peculiarly voyeuristic: every day we were asked to crowd around scantily clothed patients and scrutinise their skin. I remember being ushered in to view verrucas that had metastasised across someone's heel; to dress necrotising blisters of bullous pemphigoid (an auto-immune condition, the name of which derives from the Greek for 'pustule'); and to witness a scabies hunt that ended with the skewering of mites from tunnels in the skin of an aghast student.

One morning I was marshalled with five other students into a consulting room where a middle-aged woman in a rainbow-coloured cardigan and gypsy skirt was sitting on the side of an examination couch. Her face was haloed with blonde frizz, and she had brushed it forwards over her forehead. 'I'd like you all to see this,' said the consultant, and asked her if she'd lift up her fringe. At least two of us took a sharp intake of breath: in the centre of her forehead, just at the hairline, she was growing a horn. It was about two inches long, brown, and curling to a point like the stalk on a Halloween pumpkin.

'We're making arrangements to remove this,' said the consultant. 'These cutaneous horns are made of keratin, just like your hair, nails and ... rhinocerous horns.' Various skin conditions can generate a horn: sun-damaged skin, which may start overproducing a horny layer of skin that lengthens; some skin cancers; verrucas; and even some disorders of the sweat glands. About one in five horns turn out to be cancerous. Though of different origins, the horns are all composed of the same substance – keratin. 'They're fairly straightforward to remove,' the consultant went on, 'though this one will require a skin graft to close the defect.'

We all stood in a half-moon around her, trying not to look horrified, though the patient herself seemed unconcerned. 'Don't take it off today,' she said, and gave an impish laugh. 'I've a costume party next week – I was thinking of going as a unicorn.'

IN ROME THERE'S a statue of Moses by Michelangelo, in which he is portrayed with twinned horns, gathered brows and an intense gaze. It was commissioned for the tomb of the Renaissance pope Julius II, but sits in a small church called San Pietro in Vincoli. The horns commemorate the moment in the Bible when Moses, after receiving the ten commandments, descends Mount Sinai to his people with his face noticeably changed. St Jerome, in translating the Hebrew into Latin, described the transformation of his face as 'horned', and ever since, in the iconography of the West, that's how Moses has been represented. The Moses of Michelangelo is an enthralling, masterful piece of sculpture

– Sigmund Freud devoted a lengthy and breathless essay to it ('How often have I mounted the steep steps ... and have essayed to support the angry scorn of the hero's glance!')

Transformations in the classical as well as the Biblical tradition tend to imply an element of divine justice: in the *Metamorphoses* of Apuleius someone behaving like an ass becomes a donkey, in the *Metamorphoses* of Ovid a blood-thirsty murderer changes into a wolf. The Bible has a couple of horned transformations: in Deuteronomy 33 there's a prophet whose horns convey strength and grandeur, while the book of Revelation is stuffed with horned messengers from hell. What meaning or justice was served by putting horns onto Moses's head?

Three and a half centuries ago the physician and poly-math Thomas Browne puzzled over this inconsistency, and so went back to the Bible's original Hebrew and Greek. He realised that in Hebrew the word 'kaeran' means 'glorified' or 'shining' and that the almost identical 'karan' means 'horned', and concluded that the western iconography of Moses, for more than a millennium, is all down to a mis-translation. Horns, Browne concedes, are the 'hieroglyphic of authority, power and dignity' and so of all the transfor-mations that could have been effected on the face of Moses these were perhaps not inappropriate.* In Ovid, the future king of Rome accepts his destiny only when horns start growing from his skull. The confusion between 'horned' and 'shining' too is an ancient one – Browne quotes the Roman philosopher Macrobius: 'The Libyans reckon their god Hammon to be the setting sun, and they portray him with ram's horns, since these are the source of that animal's strength, as sunbeams are of the sun's.'

---

* Attila the Hun and Alexander the Great were generally depicted with horned helmets. In the Qur'an, Alexander is referred to simply as the 'Two-Horned One', *Dhul-Qarnayn*.

FREUD'S PSYCHOANALYSIS takes it for granted that the emanations and irritations of skin can reflect aspects of our inner life – almost as if the skin can be a barometer of our mental and emotional weather. In the early years of the twentieth century more pedestrian skin complaints like eczema and even nettle rash were assumed to be reactions to psychological or emotional conflicts. Many of my own patients notice that their psoriasis and eczema worsen during periods of anxiety or poor sleep – an observation that modern theories of immunobiology struggle to explain. Modern medicine is fairly good at knowing how to subdue skin diseases when they flare up, but our knowledge of what kindles them in the first place remains embarrassingly poor.

If skin can be a barometer to psychic weather, so too can hair – as a reaction to an emotional shock it's well known to turn white or fall out. In medical journals, this phenomenon is called 'Marie Antoinette syndrome', because of the widespread belief that the French queen's hair blanched over a single night, waiting for the gallows. Over a century ago Leonard Landois wrote,

> One of the oldest problems of pathology and physiology which has escaped scientific research and is still clouded in mythical darkness is the sudden whitening of the hair. I call it a mythical darkness, because the reports, dating mostly from older times, sound more like fairy tales than scientific observations.

But it's no fairy tale: modern dermatologists have confirmed it. Once a strand of hair leaves its follicle within the scalp it's dead – it can't change colour unless bleached. But the phenomenon of sudden whitening happens not through a change in the pigment, but through the preferential shedding of coloured hair after a fright or a shock, leaving only pale hairs behind. No one understands why the immune system attacks coloured hair in this way, and there is no known treatment.

The first historical example is in the Talmud, when bereavement is described as greying the hair. Inconsolable grief whitened the hair of Shah Jahan following the death of his wife Mumtaz Mahal (unassuaged by the building of her mausoleum, the Taj Mahal). The grief doesn't have to be for loved ones – the loss of books can do it too. On hearing of the loss of his ship with numerous priceless manuscripts, the hair of the Renaissance scholar Guarino of Verona turned white. There are numerous examples in the literature of hair-whitening following imprisonment awaiting execution: Ludovico Sforza, when captured by King Ludwig of France; Sir Thomas More in the Tower of London; and a military officer called D'Alben in pre-revolutionary France (whose hair blanched only down one side, the right). The *Chronique d'Arras* tells of the hair-whitening of a condemned criminal at the court of Charles V, and Marie Antoinette has her Scottish counterpart in Mary Queen of Scots, whose hair may have turned white awaiting execution (or it may just have been that she had more grey hair than she was ordinarily willing to admit). Of Mary's execution Stefan Zweig wrote:

> When Bulle [the executioner] wished to lift the head by the hair and show it to those assembled, he gripped only the wig, and the head dropped onto the ground. It rolled like a ball across the scaffold and when the executioner stooped once more to seize it, the onlookers could discern that it was that of an old woman with close-cropped and grizzled hair.

HORNS DON'T JUST SIGNIFY DIGNITY, but also lust, gaiety and mischief. They are the symbols of stag parties, infidelity and inexperience (greenhorns). Pan, the Greek god of shepherds and sex, had two horns, as did Bacchus, the god of wine and of fertility. 'There be many Unicorns', wrote Sir Thomas Browne, 'and consequently many Horns … Since what Horns soever they be that pass among us, they are not the Horns of one, but several animals.' As a medical student I was warned against the temptation of jumping to obscure, dramatic diagnoses – if I heard hoof-beats, I was instructed to think of horses not zebras, and never mind the possibility of unicorns. Though he accepted that a variety of species could be unicornous, Thomas Browne doesn't mention human unicorns and likely never met one. Since that afternoon in Dermatology clinic, neither have I.

But preserved in the anatomical collections of the University of Edinburgh is the horn of a human unicorn: Elizabeth Low. The stories behind many of the specimens in the collection have been lost over the centuries, but Low's is preserved thanks to a silver medallion attached to the horn itself. The horn began growing in 1664, the year that Browne was elected a Fellow of the College of Physicians. It was removed in 1671, the year Browne was knighted.

'This horn was cut by Arthur Temple', it reads, 'Chirurgeon, out of the head of Elizabeth Low, being three inches above the right ear, before thir witnesses Andrew Temple,

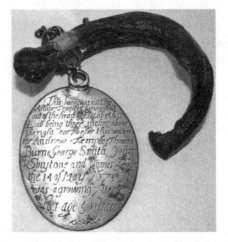

Thomas Burne, George Smith, John Smyton and James Twedie, the 14 of May 1671. It was agrowing 7 years, her age 50 years.'

FOR CENTURIES, it's been assumed that Michelangelo's Moses depicts the moment when the prophet catches the Israelites in the act of worshipping a golden calf, and his expression is one of incandescent fury. In defence of this perspective Freud quotes two contemporaries, Henry Thode and Carl Justi, in describing Moses's face as 'a mixture of wrath, pain and contempt'; 'quivering with horror and pain'. In Rome once I went to see Moses's face, and he didn't look angry to me – but wary, astonished, and even a bit frightened. It's true his eyebrows are gathered, but the left one slopes downwards, and his expression seems more a backward glance than a furious stare, as if he can't quite wrench his gaze from something terrifying or even wondrous.

There's an alternative view: the statue might just commemorate an earlier moment in the story, when Moses has

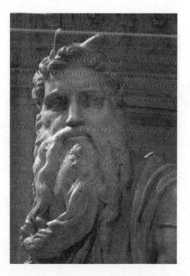

asked God to reveal himself. His face would show not anger, but heaven-struck, terrified awe. It's one of the strangest and most powerful scenes in the Hebrew Bible – it's hard to think of a more fitting moment for Michelangelo to immortalise. It's just a pity that, being sculpted in marble, we can't tell if Moses's hair has turned white.

7

Birth: Reshaping the Heart

When brought to birth, man is not yet completed; he must be born a second time.

Mircea Eliade, *The Sacred and the Profane*

THE FIRST BABY I delivered was at the end of a long night shift as a medical student. Her parents had arrived on the ward the previous afternoon, when the mother was still in the first stage of labour. We were formal and polite with one another at first – this was their first baby, and they knew it to be my first delivery – but after hours of blood and shit and sweat we were like old friends. Long after I'd qualified, every year on her birthday, I'd receive in the post a photo of their little girl. Whenever I went travelling I'd send her postcards.

I remember my hands shaking as I held her in those first moments, silenced by a sense of wonder. She took her first gasps; to watch her body change from a pallid blue to pink was like seeing colour return to a landscape after an eclipse. We were on an upper floor of a rural Scottish hospital, and the summer sunrise cast golden light on the bare institutional walls. I took a towel to dry her, clamped the cord when it stopped pulsing, and passed her up to her mother. She cried out, and I was stopped short by a tiny, powerful voice that until moments before hadn't existed.

I have attended many births since hers, and my sense of amazement has never greyed at new life, new breath, claiming its place in the world. It's glorious to see colour and life flooding into new limbs, to watch a baby join the cavalcade of life thanks to a concert of changes in the heart.

THE HEART BEGINS as two rolled tubes on a flat embryonic disc, which coalesce to form a bulbous sac that twists and knots as it grows – a fattening snake folding itself into the basket of the ribs.

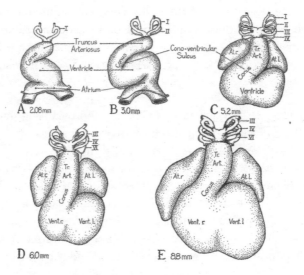

We speak of 'the circulation' but in reality human beings have two: a 'pulmonary circulation' for our lungs, and a 'systemic circulation' for the rest. The ventricle on the right pumps to the lungs, the ventricle on the left pumps to everywhere else, and the two beat simultaneously. Every beat of an adult heart pushes about seventy millilitres in tandem into each circulation; the two bloodstreams cross at the heart in an endlessly flowing figure of eight. One of the many marvels of our mammalian hearts is that they manage to conduct these twinned circulations with a single pump. Another is that the baby's lungs have to develop in the absence of air to breathe – the foetus gets all its oxygen through the placenta. Blood from the placenta gets where it's needed quickly by circumventing the baby's lungs through a pair of 'shunts': ingenious channels which shift blood from the right-sided pulmonary circulation to the left-sided systemic circulation.

The first shunt is a hole between the right atrium and the left, the 'foramen ovale'. Oxygen-enriched blood courses from the placenta, through the umbilical cord, and into the largest vein of the body. This vein is fluted at just such an angle that about a third of its blood, on entering the right side of the heart, twists straight across the atrium, through the foramen ovale, and onto the left side of the heart, where it can take oxygenated blood out to the brain and torso where it's needed. In my summers as an anatomist I'd seek out this window with astonishment: the hearts we dissected were of men and women who'd lived into old age, and yet the impression left by the foramen ovale was still visible, as was the groove in the atrial wall that rolled and directed blood towards it. To examine the walls of the adult right atrium is to see foetal fluid dynamics imprinted in the heart.*

The second shunt necessary for life in the womb is the 'ductus arteriosus', a fat trunk of a vessel that spills 90 per cent of the volume of every heartbeat away from the lungs and into the aorta. This channel is also fluted at a very particular angle, calibrated to draw bluer, more deoxygenated

---

* In about 15 to 30 per cent of us the foramen ovale stays patent into adulthood (a 'PFO'). William Harvey, the discoverer of the circulation of the blood, thought PFOs might permit their owners to breathe underwater. He was wrong: PFOs make diving more dangerous. They permit gas bubbles that form in the blood on surfacing to cross from the right circulation to the left, where they may cause strokes in the brain.

blood from the right ventricle down the descending aorta, and out to the placenta to be re-oxygenated.

Human babies start out in the earliest weeks of pregnancy with tails, and gill arches at their throats like fish. The heart develops in the throat from the vessels of these gill arches. As the embryo grows, its heart migrates down from the neck to its place in the chest. As it descends it remains connected to its original nerve supply in the neck, which is why for many people, the only sign of a heart attack is that they feel a pain in the throat and jaw. The closure of the ductus is a transformation essential to sustain our air-breathing lives, part of the transformation that turns a blue newborn pink.

All large arteries have a layer of muscle between the inner and outer coats, but the ductus is special: it has a double spiral of opposing helical fibres. It's the contraction of these fibres that closes the vessel off after birth, and they're triggered to do it by sensing oxygen from the baby's first gasps. If that early closure fails, the blood flow in the ductus reverses, damaging the lungs and overexerting the heart.

The Greek physician Galen didn't know about those helical fibres, but made a surprisingly accurate observation of ductus closure two millennia ago:

> The ductus joining the aorta to the pulmonary artery not only ceases to grow after birth, when all the other parts of the animal are growing, but it can be seen to become thinner and thinner, until as time progresses, it dries up completely and wears away.

In the dissection room I'd find its remnants: frayed scraps of fibrous tissue under the arch of the aorta, and marvel that they were all that was left of a once broad, vigorous conduit of blood.

A ductus that hasn't closed by seventy-two hours after birth gets classified as a 'patent ductus arteriosus' or PDA, and can be dangerous. 'Failure of the ductus arteriosus to close shortly after birth is associated with significant neonatal morbidity and mortality,' concluded a recent review; 'Early diagnosis is essential.'

I'M ACCUSTOMED TO LISTENING to the hearts of newborns: every baby born to a patient of my practice is seen soon after birth. The heart of a newborn beats more quickly than that of an adult – at least double the speed – the two pairs of valves making a rapid, see-saw staccato as they close in unison at more than two beats a second. There's something fragile about it, but vital; I'm acutely conscious that I'm hearing the first few beats of a heart that will beat billions of times – with luck, long after my own has fallen silent.

A decade after making that first delivery, a baby just a few weeks old was brought to my clinic for a check-up. His mother, Joy, told me 'He's not feeding very well.' 'He's trying,' she said, 'but it's as if he can't coordinate sucking with breathing. And his nose is getting blocked up.' She stretched the baby's tiny body out on her lap; a river-map of veins showed through translucent abdominal skin. His eyes blinked unseeing from that half-womb half-world that babies occupy in the first weeks of life. I asked about the birth: Connor had been born a week or two early, and there had been no complications. At first he'd thrived, and regained his birth weight, and when I plotted out his size on a growth chart I saw that he was around the 90th centile – meaning that only 10 per cent of babies his age would be larger. At first he'd fed well, but for a few days now he'd been struggling.

I warmed the end of the stethoscope by rubbing it on my hand, knelt on the floor, and put it to Connor's ribs. Instead of a soft staccato there was a legato, each beat joined to the next by a muffled rumble, loudest to the left side of his breastbone, and audible, though quieter, along his back. His lungs sounded healthy, with plenty of free passage of air. 'He has a murmur,' I said, taking the stetho-scope from his chest. Joy's eyes widened, her nostrils flared a little, her head became very still on her neck. 'He's not feeding so well because his nose is blocked, but I'd like to have his heart checked too. Lots of babies have murmurs – it's usually nothing to worry about.'

'Could it be serious?' she asked, searching my face as much as she listened to my words.

'Not necessarily' – I tried to look relaxed – 'we'll need an ultrasound scan of his heart to know more.'

As I typed up a referral letter Joy buckled him into a sling with grim efficiency; as she left down the clinic corridor I heard her call her husband on the phone. A couple of weeks later a letter from the paediatric cardiolo-gist arrived.

'Thank you for referring this infant, in whom you noted a murmur,' it said. 'There is no family history of valvular heart disease, though a grandfather had a persistent ductus arte-riosus closed as an adolescent.' The cardiologist had plotted Connor's weight as I'd done, checked all of his pulses, and noted that when she placed a hand over Connor's chest, she could feel a transmitted impulse from the left ventricle of the heart – beating more vigorously than it should.

As Connor's heart had knotted into position it had left one thread untied – a patent ductus. 'It is unlikely this will now close on its own,' the cardiologist added, 'and we may need to arrange surgical ligation at around six months, or transcatheter occlusion.'

The next time I saw Joy was in the clinic corridor a couple of months later, when her son was four months old. She had just had him weighed: he was still growing along the 90th centile with regard to his length, but his weight had dropped to the 50th, because he was getting slimmer. 'Sometimes I can even hear his murmur,' she said. 'Do you think there's a chance it'll close on its own?'

I did my best to reassure her, but by the next appointment

with the paediatricians his weight had dropped to the 35th centile. They assured Joy that Connor's heart hadn't sustained any irreversible damage, though it was now a little wider than it should have been, and the lungs were showing signs of strain. The cardiologists wanted to see whether it would close further on its own.

The day of his 'cardiac catheterisation' Connor was anaesthetised, and a narrow tube was introduced from an easily accessible blood vessel in his leg up and into his heart. Pressures in the pulmonary arteries and aorta were measured and compared. By then his weight had fallen to the 25th centile, and his length had begun to fall off too. Sometimes a patent ductus arteriosus has a shape that means it can be closed from within, using only wires introduced down the catheterisation tubes, but Connor's could not. His surgery was two days later.

The next time I saw him was the following week. He fed from Joy's left breast, and she lifted up his vest to show me the scar where the surgeons had cut into the left side of his chest. They had splayed open his ribs, collapsed his lung, and with a watchmaker's precision, tied off the ductus.

'The noise has gone,' Joy said, 'you can't feel his heart thudding through his chest any more. He's feeding better too. Who'd have thought a tiny thread, tied in exactly the right place, could make such a difference?'

Three months later Connor was back up to the 50th centile in terms of his weight, and his chest X-ray showed that his heart had reverted to normal size. The return of his growth was dramatic: at a year his weight had returned to the 90th centile. 'Connor can now be regarded as having a completely normal heart,' said the final letter discharging him from clinic. 'Looking to the future, there is no need for him to take any precautions whatsoever.'

THE CHARACTERISTIC MURMUR of a patent ductus was first described over a century ago by a Dr George Gibson, a few hundred yards away from my clinic in Edinburgh. A physician in the city's Royal Infirmary, Gibson described the distinctive 'thrill' he felt over the chest as blood rumbled through the ductus. Turbulence in an artery causes its inner lining to roughen, the way a river abrades its banks. That abraded layer is fertile soil for seedlings of bacteria to lodge and grow. Until a few decades ago, children with patent ductus often died from these infections, or from the failure of an overexerted heart.

Until 1938, children with a patent ductus had to live with it, or more often die with it, but that year at the Boston Children's Hospital a surgeon managed to close one. His name was Robert Gross, and his achievement is all the more astonishing given that he had the use of only one eye. He practised the minuscule stereoscopic movements required by dismantling and reassembling watches. Closing the ductus was considered so risky that Gross did it surreptitiously, when his boss went away on holiday. Only two surgeons had tried before him: one had opened the chest to find no ductus present (before ultrasound was invented, misdiagnosis was common), and the other proved technically impossible – the child died soon afterwards. 'The child or youth who possesses a patent ductus faces an uncertain future,' wrote Gross, 'like Damocles, he leads a precarious existence, never knowing when he might be cut down by the danger which menaces him.'

Gross's first patient was a sickly child who had narrowly survived to the age of seven. His account of the surgical innovation, published in the *Annals of Surgery*, describes a wan, melancholy girl: 'Frequently she would stand still, have a rather frightened appearance, and place her hand over her heart. When asked what was the trouble she would whisper "Something wrong inside of here."' She couldn't play with the other children, and her mother often reported a frightening buzzing noise coming from deep within her chest.

Gross was convinced that this devastating problem had a simple, technical solution. First he went to the dissection room, where, working on cadavers, he figured out the best place to open the ribcage to get at the ductus.

Then he trialled his procedure on a series of living, anaesthetised dogs, until he was confident he had perfected the procedure of dissecting the pulsing aortic arch away from the pulmonary arteries. It took 'great care and patience,' he said: 'in a small place between the great vessels ... space is at a premium'. There was a risk of damaging three nerves: one that sustains the breath, one that coordinates digestion and pulse rate, and one that supplies the larynx – a scalpel-slip could induce suffocation, or make his patient mute. 'I have spent as long as an hour in locating, freeing up, and tracing this nerve, for it is time well spent,' he wrote of the nerve to the larynx; 'once it is brought into view, the remainder of the dissection seems to be on a safer and surer basis.' After a meticulous clearing of the fibrous tissue around the ductus, he recommended pinching it closed for several minutes before proceeding. 'If no undesirable effects are produced ... the ductus may be permanently ligated.' This he did with heavy braided silk, which had to be 'drawn up *very tightly* if complete obliteration is to be effected'. The linings of his patient's lung were sutured up again, her lung re-expanded, and after a day resting in bed, she was allowed up in a wheelchair.

Gross's first paper describes four separate cases, all achieved without complications. His technique had brought a transformation to the heart and the great vessels that, in most of us, occurs naturally in the first hours after birth. 'The child's general condition has been excellent,' he wrote of one of the cases. 'She has returned to school and in the first two months after operation she has gained three pounds in weight.' A length of silk, expertly tied, had effected a kind of rebirth.

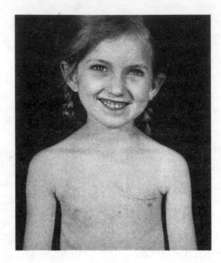

8

Rejuvenation: An Alchemy of Youth and Beauty

Whereat Hecabe ... leapt into the sea and changed her aged form.

Nicander's *Heteroeumena* ('Beings Made Alien')

IN MIKHAIL BULGAKOV'S NOVEL *The Master and Margarita* there's a scene of miraculous rejuvenation, accomplished by a magical cream. Margarita Nikolayevna, a thirty-year-old woman, is sitting on a bench in Moscow's Alexander Gardens beneath the Kremlin when a suspicious fang-toothed man (later revealed as an agent of Satan) presents her with a golden casket, heavy and ornate as a reliquary. He tells her to wait until exactly half past eight that evening before opening it and applying the contents to her skin. For reasons too complicated to summarise, she agrees.

At 8.29 p.m. Margarita can't wait any longer: she lifts the heavy box of gold and opens the lid. The cream is yellowish and oily, and gives off the aroma of earth, marshland and forest. She begins rubbing it into her forehead and cheeks, where it is absorbed quickly and greaselessly, producing a tingling effect over her skin. Then she looks in the mirror and drops the casket in shock.

Her eyes have changed colour to green, and her eyebrows have grown from narrow, plucked lines into perfect, symmetrical arcs. A worry-line between them has vanished. Shadows around her temples, and 'barely detectable sets of crowsfeet' have vanished. The skin of her cheeks begins to glow pink, her forehead becomes pale and perfectly smooth, and the artificial waves in her hair are loosened into flowing and natural-looking curls. She laughs with glee, throws off her bathrobe, and begins to rub the cream all over her naked body. A tense headache that had bothered her since her meeting in the gardens disappears, her arms and legs grow stronger and firmer. Jumping into the air with joy, she sinks slowly and elegantly back to earth, as if being lowered by angels. The cream has granted her the power of flight.

Bulgakov was trained as a doctor and his book brims with vivid clinical details: of blood spurting at a beheading, of a gently persuasive psychiatric interrogation, of the grinding crunch of a leg being severed. He brings the same attentiveness to the effects of the cream.

As a physician, he must have known that creams in the real world can only slow the inevitable process of ageing, never reverse it. To keep skin looking youthful, it's more important what you *avoid* than what you rub on: smoking, unhealthy food and sun exposure all add years to the skin. Once its natural elasticity has started to fade, there's no cream on earth that can restore it.

IT WAS AN AIRPORT, but it could have been a shopping mall, a railway station or even a hospital concourse anywhere in the rich world: strip lighting, cathedral-high ceilings, gantries of air ducts, wear-resistant carpets, overpriced cafés, gallimaufries of shops, and target demographics idling on uncomfortable chairs. The products for sale vary slightly with the season, but not much: magazines, gifts, clothes and bags; caffeine, electronics, junk food and alcohol. A solitary chemist's shop offers a different promise, with illuminated banners of 'health' and 'beauty'. But what they are really selling is youth.

Medieval alchemists had a thousand different names for youth elixirs, and the contemporary rejuvenation industry is not far behind. The first three creams I picked up belonged to the same range, and blended an appetising list of ingredients: rosemary, chamomile, cocoa, eucalyptus, borage, avocado, echinacea, aloe vera, hops, cucumber, calendula, and 'heavenly fragrance of rose-scented geranium'. On another shelf, an exotic melon from the Kalahari had been rarefied and liquefied, and presented for application to heat-damaged hair. There were seductive promises of rejuvenated and radiant-looking skin. One of the creams promised a transformative reduction in the appearance of fine lines and wrinkles, and another a 'firmer, lifted, and youthful-looking complexion'. There were variably blended products customised for hands, nails, feet, face, body and breast. Some creams were described as 'precious serums', the application of which was not just beneficial, but necessary. Each offered to make skin 'visibly plumper, smoother and rejuvenated'.

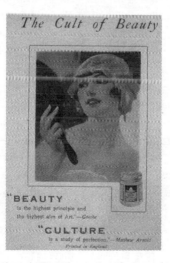

The men's shelf ran to just four products, which in their own way also promised youth, though their effects were described as calming, softening and smoothing rather than rejuvenating (as if mollifying male character, not male skin, was their object). The divergent marketing approach for men's products was replicated on the shelves stocking vitamin supplements, which promised youth and improved complexion for women, but strength and potency for men. These were advertised as being necessary not just for health, but to confer 'vitality'.

The story of Bulgakov's Margarita is part of a long tradition, from Snow White's wicked stepmother (who wanted to remain 'fairest of them all') to the Germanic legends that granted vigorous youth to men heroic enough to slay a dragon. There's a spectacular example of youth enchantment in Ovid's *Metamorphoses* when Jason defeats a dragon to get hold of a golden fleece, then implores his wife – the sorceress Medea – to rejuvenate his father Aeson, using a potion of herbs so exotic they could have been taken from a modern cosmetics catalogue. In her dragon-harnessed chariot Medea makes a tour of the most glamorous and outlandish sites in the Greek world in order to gather herbs. She fills twinned holes in the earth with the blood of a sacrificed sheep, adds wine and milk, then dips flaming torches in before setting them ablaze. Into a cauldron go roots from Thessaly, sands from Oceanus at the earth's limit, and powdered rocks from the far east.*

Medea used a desiccated old olive wand to stir the brew; as she did so it sprouted leaves then grew heavy with olives. Spatters from the broth caused flowers and grass to spring up on the cold dark earth. At this final sign Medea felt ready to proceed: she slit Aeson's jugular veins and poured in her potion. 'Quickly his beard and his hair lost their whiteness ... New flesh filled out his sagging wrinkles,

---

* Chinese alchemists traditionally mixed and heated different minerals, not herbs, to create youth treatments, and it's as if Ovid was aware of Chinese preference.

and his limbs grew young and strong. The old king mar-
velled at the change in himself, recalling that this was the
Aeson of forty years ago.'

BETH LORD WAS in her mid-fifties and wore elegant designer
suits and blusher on her cheeks. Her vigilant eyes were heavy
with mascara, and her eyebrows were as delicately contoured
as the finest sable paintbrush. She'd trained as a lawyer but
hadn't worked for years. Her husband was an executive at
an investment bank, and worked long periods away between
offices in New York and Shanghai. 'About twenty years ago
he told me "we don't need the money" and encouraged me
to quit. So I did.' At first, she didn't miss work, being a busy
mother of a young daughter, and she signed up for every
school and local committee that asked her to contribute.
In addition to her rounds of meetings and school fairs she
attended a gym every day, and started a small-scale business
selling cosmetics to friends and neighbours.

Usually in clinic we talked about her anxiety, which was
high, and her mood, which was low, as well as her struggles
to relate to her husband. They hadn't had sex for years,
and she would sometimes ask me to recommend relationship counsellors, or how to improve her libido, as well as
that of her husband. My advice never seemed to reap much
reward. One day she attended complaining of chest pains,
which had been gripping her ribcage at night – usually when
her husband was away. She was anxious that they might
be coming from her heart, or from some cosmetic breast
surgery she'd had in the past.

'I didn't know you'd had surgery,' I said, glancing at
her notes on the screen. She unbuttoned her blouse and
pulled down her bra to show the circumferential scars at the
periphery of each nipple, where the disc of tissue had been
resected and repositioned higher on the breast. 'It hasn't
given me any problems up to now,' she said, 'do you think
those operations could be causing the pain?' Each silvered

circle radiated a thin line, which dropped down over the recontoured breast – invisible in dim light but shown up by the examination lamps. 'I had it done ten years ago.'

I told her that it was unlikely her pains were caused by scarring. 'Did you ever have any other operations?' I asked. We had never discussed plastic surgery.

'Oh, a couple, but you won't have the records – it's all been done abroad,' she said. 'I've had Botox around the eyes, some fat at the top of my arms taken out, and – oh! Some sagging skin taken off my belly.' She indicated another circular scar around her navel where the skin had been pulled taut and trimmed, then repositioned over her umbilicus. 'That was just to deal with the stretch marks after being pregnant with Margaret.'

Her daughter Margaret suffered from migraines, and I'd come to know her a little over the years. 'How *is* Margaret?' I asked.

'Fine, fine,' she said with a quick, nervous smile. 'She's off at college now, having a ball. I'm happy she's away, you know, living her own life.' But her voice suggested otherwise, and the fingers of her right hand fretted at the diamonds on her left.

There were a few tests to arrange, to confirm that the pain wasn't coming from Beth's heart. Its character and timing implied it wasn't coming from her lungs, ribs or past surgery. 'You know, much of the time we can't find any physical cause for chest pains,' I told her. 'The pains come and go on a rhythm that's more to do with worries or anxieties than anything else. When those worries and anxieties ease, so does the pain.' We talked a little about breathing techniques to try the next time she felt the pain.

'Sometimes,' I added, 'these kinds of pains can be your mind and your body's way of telling you that something in your life has to change. It won't let you rest until that happens.'

'My life could do with a few changes,' she said.

THE EARLIEST KNOWN TEXT concerned with the elixirs of youth is an early Chinese commentary on the *I Ching*, the 'Book of Changes', in which chemical substances and processes are tentatively correlated with the book's famous hexagrams. The *I Ching* takes it for granted that the universe and all beings in it are caught up in cycles of transformation, and suggests that the astute application of mystical and medical knowledge can influence those changes for the better.

In Europe, alchemists were obsessed with generating gold, but in China they preferred to work on youth elixirs. A string of Chinese alchemists claimed to have created a rejuvenating potion; Joseph Needham, the historian, scientist and Sinologist, was so struck by the frequency with which Chinese emperors were poisoned by these drugs that he tabulated a list of victims. In around 300 CE, a Chinese alchemist called Ko Hung collated various recipes. Three centuries later a more detailed treatise specified the inclusion of obscure, exotic substances such as mercurial salts and compounds of sulphur. There are over a thousand different names for these potions, most of which carried the same basic mineral ingredients.

One of Ko Hung's near-contemporaries in the West, a Byzantine called Synesius, believed that the physical transformations effected by alchemy were less important than the mental positions adopted by its practitioners. A true alchemy of youth didn't require a laboratory or precious, exotic substances; all that was needed was the right kind of incantation, and a change in attitude.

'I'VE LEFT HIM,' Beth told me when she next came to clinic. 'Or rather, he's left me, or we've both left each other – either way, the marriage is over.' There was a fierce and triumphant gleam in her eye that I hadn't seen before. Though she was still meticulous about her clothes I noticed she was without her usual layers of make-up. She looked fired-up, vital, and slightly in shock.

'What happened?'

'I've known for years that something had to change ...' she began. 'Maybe I just held on for the sake of Margaret. But those chest pains, they were the last straw.'

One night she'd felt the pains beginning, and rather than worry over them she'd got up out of bed, put the lights on, and had written out a list of every disappointment and frustration in her life. 'It was quite a list,' she said, with a wry smile. 'Two sides of paper. But one thing kept coming up again and again – the sense of being trapped in this marriage, trapped with a man who had lost interest in me and in our life together. And the worry that time's running out.'

'So what did you do?' I asked.

'When he came back from business last time, I showed him the list.'

'And?'

'He's been having an affair for years! He admitted it! With a woman twenty years younger than me.'

I waited for a few moments.

'It was almost a relief to hear him confess,' she said. 'Well, I'm better off now without him. That's the first change, but there'll be more.'

'What do you think you'll do next?' I asked.

'He told me I didn't need to work ... but we all need work, don't we? And I want to travel!'

'How has Margaret taken the news?'

She beamed back at me with pride: 'That was the greatest surprise of all,' she said. '"Mum, you should have done it years ago," she told me.'

BULGAKOV WROTE THAT Margarita felt 'anointed' by the magical cream: a glorious sense of freedom ran through her limbs, her body fizzed with giddy pleasure. She had the sudden conviction that she would leave her home and her husband, who she did not love, and begin a new life.

After shouting 'Hurray for the cream!' to no one in particular, she flies through the air to her husband's desk and, without hesitation or deliberation, writes a note asking him to forget her.

A sound disturbs her – a broomstick knocking in the cupboard. Margarita opens its door, jumps onto the broomstick, and zooms naked out of the window. Magic has rendered her invisible to onlookers – it's understood that this youthful beauty is for her own pleasure, not anyone else's. After taunting her boring neighbour, taking revenge on an enemy, she takes off on a flight out of Moscow.

At first she flies at tremendous speed across the Russian landscape, her toes brushing the tops of trees, the great rivers of Siberia passing beneath her so quickly that a strobe of reflected moonlight flashes beneath her feet. Then she slows to enjoy her new perspective, and 'savour the thrill of flight'.

MEDICAL PRACTICE IS so thick with daily revelations, so deeply textured with the intimacies and details of so many lives, that several months went by before I realised I hadn't seen Beth Lord again. She must have moved away, given up on her prescriptions of antidepressants, or had no need of the space our consultations offered. Sometimes a therapeutic relationship comes to an end because it has achieved its aim, and sometimes because a stray phrase has caused offence. Usually I never find out why.

A couple of years later I saw Beth's name again on my clinic list. I called her name from the waiting-room door; 'Long time no see,' she said, rising quickly from her seat and striding after me to the office.

'So how have you been?' I asked.

She was still gracefully dressed, but wore little make-up, and the expression around her eyes was cheerful and relaxed. In her attitude and her appearance she seemed younger. 'Fine, marvellous really,' she said, taking her seat.

'When we last met you spoke about leaving your husband ...'

'And I did!' she finished with glee. 'And I took off travelling. I've been twice around the world since then ...'

9

Tattooing: The Art of Transformation

They were stains of some sort or other ... And what is it, thought I, after all! It's only his outside; a man can be honest in any sort of skin.

Herman Melville, *Moby Dick*

IT'S THIN, THE BARRIER that separates us from the world — when I see skin blister or crack I'm often startled by just how insubstantial it is. The subtlest of scratches may leave a scar; the most trivial of abrasions may drive dirt under the skin and leave a permanent stain. The first tattoos must have been like this, unintentional, ash or mud forced into the body through falls or flint wounds.

A few years ago I had a clinical attachment to a medical research unit in East Africa. One of the local doctors, Faith, took care of me. She had trained in Nairobi, was efficient and imperturbable, and her long, braided hair was knotted high on her head. As she led me on her rounds she spoke of her grief at the corruption that robbed funds from the hospital. One of the hundreds of bedside stops we made together was to a malnourished boy, about eight years old, who lay face down on a dirty bed. He had cerebral palsy, had fallen in a fire, and before coming to the hospital had been nursed at home with inadequate, dirty dressings. Mottled burn scars made a chiaroscuro of his back; pressure sores too, some infected. Embedded in the burn scars were flecks of charcoal that would be almost impossible now to remove – if he survived, he'd carry their marks for the rest of his life. 'He is improving a little,' said Faith, her voice matter-of-fact as she picked up his chart. 'When I admitted him I almost cried, he had been so neglected. But then I remember that I don't care. I can't.'

For accommodation I rented a bungalow in an empty holiday complex near the hospital. One day the manager's ex-husband arrived, sacked the staff, switched off the water supply and locked the main gate. For a couple of days I had to wash my clothes and dishes in the pool, until I found a room in another house with some colleagues, further away from the hospital but next to the beach. It was a round house, surrounded by the bush, open to the air and with iron bars instead of walls, and it came with a resident population of giant millipedes, dive-bomber beetles, and smug, fat geckos. Within the toilet rim lived a colony of tiny frogs, naturally selected to swim fast enough to avoid being flushed away.

At night I'd hear the sounds of partying carry through the trees from the house next door. The neighbours at that time were Samburu warriors from the highlands of Kenya. They had recently been the subject of a documentary, and had come down to the coast to celebrate with the film's director. At an evening party I was taken aside by one of the men: he didn't like it down by the Indian Ocean he told me – too hot, too many people, and the locals ate too much fish. No self-respecting Samburu would eat such food. It was different in his homeland, he said: cool, spacious, healthy, and a hunter could eat red meat all year round.

Around his thighs he had a pattern of circular scars: raised, shiny blebs as if divots of flesh had been prised out with thorns, then left to heal. I asked how he had got them. 'It's done with burning sticks,' he said; 'we do it when we become *moran*, warriors.' He ran his fingers over the scars, remembering. 'For days afterwards it was very hard to walk.' The whorled patterns of the markings were like fingerprints writ large. Others on his trunk were arranged in neat cubic geometries, like *I Ching* ideograms cast over the body. The young men in his tribe were all marked this way, he said, before they were expected to go out to fight against neighbouring tribes, such as the Turkana.

'Did you ever fight the Turkana?' I asked.

He shook his head. 'They are near to Somalia. They have AK-47s.'

He'd visited Edinburgh once for the film festival. 'Very cold', he remembered. I imagined this African warrior, skin like polished anthracite, scars hidden beneath blue jeans, bracing himself against the icy brine of the North Sea wind.

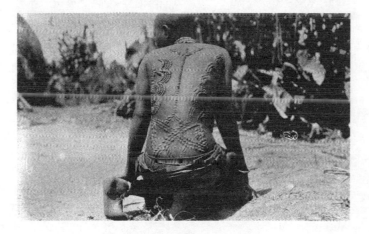

IN MY CLINIC in Edinburgh I often see another kind of scarification – the 'deliberate self-harm' of those who cut themselves in moments of intense anguish. I asked one of my patients, Calvin, how he'd fallen into the habit: 'It started in secret,' he said, 'something I did in my own bedroom. I'd take a razor, or unscrew the blade from a pencil sharpener, and just nick the skin ever so slightly. Just enough to draw blood. I'd catch the blood in tissues, then smuggle the dirty tissues out to a bin far from the house. It made me feel better, for a while. But then worse, you know, afterwards.'

'Where did you cut yourself?' I asked.

'At first just here' – he pointed to his hip – 'so that if I was wearing shorts no one would be able to see the scars.'

Calvin pulled down the waistband of his trousers and half-stood to show me: a marbled lattice of white lines overlay his hip.

'And then?'

'Then it wasn't enough – I switched to the other hip, and then my forearms. At the beginning I thought I could just wear long sleeves, and then I didn't care any more. Something switched in me – I *wanted* others to see the scars. I wanted my mum, my dad, my teachers, everyone around me to see how unhappy I was.'

We were both silent for a few seconds. 'What do you think about them now?' I asked.

'For a long time I was happy to have them. That phase in my life is past, but it's a big part of me. It's part of who I am. Those scars are a relic of my past self – I don't want to get that low again. Until recently, each time I glanced down and saw the scars, I remembered how much stronger I am these days.'

I'd been seeing Calvin for a year or so, weaning down his antidepressants slowly, checking in on the counselling and the confidence-building courses he'd signed up for. 'And now?'

'And now I'm ready to move on. I'm going to leave that part of my life behind for ever. I've decided to get tattoos, I'm going to cover them all.'

For some, the act of being tattooed is related to the same impulse to cut, but for Calvin each tattoo was a step away from the person he'd been. Over the next few visits I watched his tattoos evolve. First a Chinese dragon coiling over his left hip, flicking its tail up over the crest of his pelvis and towards his spine; 'It means vigour for me,' he said, 'a reminder that I've got hidden strength.' I looked closely – the scarring was barely noticeable. Then, a few months later, I saw him again: his right hip was overlain with a lion rampant. 'It's bold and proud, like I want to be.' Over the following year, on his right forearm, there evolved a scene of winged angels mounted on clouds, the trumpet blasts of heaven radiating around them like discharges of electricity. In the pale gaps of skin there bloomed a garden of flowers. On his left there evolved a hellish scene: ghouls, skulls and trident-bearing demons, with fanged snakeheads crammed in the spaces.

'I'm caught in the middle,' he said, pointing at his torso; 'with hell on my left side' – at this he lifted his left forearm with its ghouls and demons – 'and heaven on my right' – he lifted the angels and trumpet blasts.

'You're carrying both around with you,' I said.

'Don't we all. You must see that in your job.'

IN THE SHERLOCK HOLMES STORIES, Arthur Conan Doyle implies that the discerning detective can learn much about a person from their tattoos. 'I have made a small study of tattoo marks,' Conan Doyle has Holmes say, 'and have even contributed to the literature of the subject.' The tattoo is valued as a living testimonial to the life history of its bearer – as valuable to the physician as to the detective.

Often, when I roll up a sleeve to take blood pressure, or pull up someone's shirt to listen to their lungs, I see tattoos that ordinarily go unseen. Some are about family allegiance: the names and birthdays of children, or fidelity to a particular partner. Some tell me about military tours of duty, or time spent in the merchant navy. Tattoos of bikers, soldiers, sailors and prisoners all bear witness to membership of a closed, strictly tiered society. I remember opening a shirt to test a man's belly for appendicitis, to see his torso inscribed in a flowing copperplate: 'worrying is praying for the worst to happen'. His tattoo was a kind of self-uttered enchantment: he told me that since getting it, his lifelong anxiety had gone.

Tattoos can be helpful to the clinician in a very direct, practical way: one patient of mine could point to exactly where among a writhing sleeve of snakes to plunge a needle to be sure of getting blood. Sometimes skin is tattooed to show a radiotherapist exactly where on the body a tumour is to be targeted. Some are about forging an allegiance between the present and the future self – a lifelong keepsake of how its bearer used to be: a flower at the ankle, a rosette at the base of the spine, a cartoon character on a shoulder. And I've seen some that are emblems of transcendence and celebration: a phoenix rising from the ashes of a mastectomy scar, a garden of flowers blooming over stretch marks.

Tattooing must be among the earliest of art forms – the body as canvas, as symbol, as commemoration, as welcome, and warning. They're frameless works of art, transformations of the body surface – itself subject to ceaseless change. They break down the distinction between subject and object. Sometimes they're dismissed as something you'd get on impulse, but for most people, getting a tattoo is painful – as the poet Michael Donaghy pointed out, you'd need a 'whim of iron'. The word is Polynesian – it came into global usage with the voyages of Captain Cook, and refers to the 'tat-tat-tat' repetition of the needle as it punctures the skin (the drum roll 'tattoo' of a military band has the same origin).

It can be the puncturing of the skin that brings a tattoo to my medical attention – infections, blistering, sometimes inflammatory reactions to ink. Psychological reactions too – around half of tattoo recipients regret them. In the United States a quarter of all young and middle-aged people have a tattoo, and there are more than 100,000 tattoo-removal procedures each year. James Kern, a tattoo artist specialising in transmuting unwanted tattoos into new designs, has written: 'You will never have a happier client than someone who no longer has a tattoo that they hate. It destroys their self-esteem. I love the transformation physically and spiritually.'

Historically there have been hundreds of reasons for getting tattooed – perhaps as many reasons as there are people who have them. Anthropologists have listed a few: camouflage for hunting; to mark and propitiate puberty and pregnancy; to counteract disease; improve fertility; to mollify malign spirits. Some of the motives identified among tribal societies are just as relevant among my own patients: to take on new characteristics; to honour ancestors or descendants; to enhance one's respect among the community; to frighten enemies; to make the body a register of life events; to beautify oneself; to express an emotion (patriotism, love, friendship); to demonstrate group allegiance. Some motives seem unique to contemporary culture: as permanent facial make-up, or even to make money exhibiting yourself. I've heard of someone who tattooed his blood group onto his arm, in case he ever needed a transfusion (with an arrow pointing at the broadest vein). And there are more baleful reasons: being branded by a fascist regime; as an act of deliberate self-harm; or to relieve boredom in a prison cell.

Of the latter two, the tattoos of prisoners tell a story of bravado, isolation and violence, or affirm allegiance and status. Some prison cultures, like those in Russia or South Africa, have elaborate tattoos that symbolise crimes committed – coffins to signify a murderer, a dagger at the throat for a mercenary, wrist manacles or numerals to signify the number of years incarcerated.* For the prisoner, the body

---

* Kafka's *In The Penal Colony* describes a machine that tattoos each prisoner's body with the law that has been broken.

can be the only possession left – and the only weapon of rebellion. I've seen clumsy self-inked allegories of freedom restrained, and of gardens and birds intertwined and tangled with thorns. I've seen scrawled skulls reminiscent of the *memento mori* skeletons that dance around the borders of old gravestones. Tattoos are a way of bringing disorder, playfulness and creativity to a body living within the drudgery and order of the prison. The body in chains comes to tell a story of its own liberation.

THE FIRST I KNEW of Mark Blakewell was a sheet of paper sent in to the medical practice from the city jail: 'The above-named patient is being released from prison tomorrow,' it said, 'I'd be grateful if you would take over the methadone prescription as detailed below.' Methadone is an opiate substitute, prescribed to dull the cravings of heroin addicts. I looked up the notes we held from the time before his conviction: a catalogue of emergency department attendances for fight injuries, and a couple of psychiatric referrals that he didn't turn up to. Then a sudden silence, about ten years previously. We sent an appointment time back through to the prison nurses, and the following day he showed up in my office.

He was thin and pale, in his early forties, with crew-cut blonde hair, and tight, bloodless lips. There were lines notched into his eyebrows. He wore a green tracksuit with white stripes, and down one cheek he had twinned scars. He blinked too often, and his eyes fidgeted around the room. But the most striking thing about him was his tattoos – all amateur works, executed in thick blue ink. A spider's web was drawn up one side of his neck, and a dagger, pointing towards his heart, tattooed down the other. There were some tears tattooed onto one cheek; a loop of barbed wire circled his throat. Through his thin hair I could make out more designs on his scalp – a swastika, a skull and a Scottish flag. I glanced down at his hands: he had 'LOVE' tattooed across his right knuckles, and 'HATE' across his left. On his thumb knuckles he had clusters of blue dots, and a swallow fluttered at the web spaces between his right thumb and index finger.

He sat down next to my desk, and glowered. He had skin creases like target circles around his eyes. 'I've come for my methadone,' he said.

'Sure. What dose are you on?'

He sighed theatrically: 'If you don't know that already, you don't know what you're doing.'

'I'm just checking I've got the right details.'

'Eighty,' he said. 'And I need my Valium too.'

'Eighty, fine. But I can't give you Valium – no one comes out of prison on Valium.'

'If you think we can't get it there you really don't know what you're doing.' The consonants in his voice were hard. 'If you don't give me any, I'll have to buy it on the street. Then it'll be your fault when the police come after me.'

'If you're so nervous you have to buy street Valium, then maybe we should talk about how to ease your anxiety.'

He grunted, grabbed the prescription from my hands, and went to stand up. Then the mask of fury on his face softened, he exhaled slowly and sat down again.

'Sorry,' he said, and looked down at his shoes. He looked as if he was trying to find the words to say more.

'I'll be civil to you, if you'll be civil to me,' I said.

He sat back in his chair and took a deep breath. 'OK, let's start again.'

Each of my patients on a methadone prescription is seen monthly, and over the months, as I came to know Mark better, he grew his blonde hair long. It curled around his ears and cast the spider's web and dagger into shadow. The tattooed tears on his cheek were still prominent, and through his open-necked shirt I'd glimpse the barbed wire girdling his throat. On that first day out of prison I'd watched him manage to get his temper under control; slowly, I watched him do the same with his drug use.

One day he came in with a bandaged hand. He was wearing a polo-necked shirt, and was down from eighty to forty millilitres of methadone a day. We agreed to drop it to thirty-five. He told me he'd found a job in a mechanic's shop – a friend had recommended him for the work. 'And what happened to your hand?' I asked.

'Tattoos,' he said. 'I burned one with battery acid.'

I unwrapped the bandage: weals of reddened skin were healing over his knuckles, but blue ink was already showing through the scabs.

'They used to try this in the old days,' I said. 'They'd peel off tattooed skin, then graft new skin over the wound. It doesn't work very well – they use lasers now.'

'And does it work?' he asked.

'Sometimes,' I said. 'And your tattoos are exactly the kind it's best for. Not cheap, though.'

The lasers for tattoo removal are chosen according to the colour of pigment to be broken down – red and orange pigments need a green laser, a red laser is used for blues and blacks. It's painful too – more painful than getting the tattoo in the first place. The lasers usually lighten the skin, which can be a problem for anyone with a dark skin tone.*

I went on meeting with Mark every month, bringing his methadone down by increments – and as his addiction eased, I watched his tattoos dissolve. By the time he was at thirty millilitres a day, the tattooed tears on his cheek were just faint smudges, barely noticeable. He was living frugally, spending all of his income on the laser clinic. By twenty-five millilitres the dagger and webs at his throat were fading, and I could see he had started on the circle of barbed wire at his throat. By ten millilitres a day there

_____

* There is a push now to extend the regulation of tattoo artists to the pigments that it is legally permissible to use, in order to make them more easily removable. Bright modern pigments are the most difficult to remove with lasers.

were just blemishes to see on his face and neck, though he still had to keep his hair long enough to prevent the scalp tattoos showing through.

A year or so later I saw him in clinic again. He looked well – as he walked into my office his once grey, zipper-tight lips opened wide in a smile. He wanted me to prescribe something to help him stop smoking. I noticed the swallow still fluttered at the web space between the thumb and index finger of his right hand.

'What about that one?' I asked him, pointing down at the free-flying bird.

'That one I'm keeping,' he said.

10

Anorexia: The Enchantment of Control

This is a real illness, not a whim of spoiled rich girls. It's been treated like it's voluntary and wilful as opposed to what it is: a serious, life-threatening psychiatric and medical illness.

Diane Mickley MD

ANOREXIA NERVOSA IS AN INSCRUTABLE ILLNESS: baffling and frustrating to those who suffer it as it may be to those trying to help. Some mental illness dissolves the boundaries of the self, tearing the seams by which we hold ourselves together. Some foist on us delusions of being pursued, persecuted, contaminated – or their opposite: delusions of being powerful, grand and invulnerable. Some mental illness forces a retreat from the world, shutting down engagement in a destructive cloak of depression or catatonia. Anorexia is none of these things: a self-destructive, poisonous assault on the body and mind, a grim alliance between one of our most ancient instincts – to fast and even avoid food that we believe might harm us – and one of humanity's newer preoccupations – the way we appear to ourselves and to others.

Effective mental health therapists are part-priest and part-conjuror: they find ways to re-invoke an individual's boundaries, dissolve his or her delusions, and summon an authentic, engaged self from the shadow beneath which they've fallen. We no longer think of mental illness as a possession which descends on us, cast by powers beyond our control. Modern medical psychiatry looks at mental illness as a phenomenon of brain chemistry, but some languages still carry the sense that it comes from without as a kind of psychic weather. This perspective can be effective in neutralising any guilt or culpability a sufferer might feel – ancient physicians spoke of melancholia as something beyond our control, subject to the flux of humours, and some languages retain this sense today. There are languages in which to say 'I'm depressed' is to say 'a sadness is on me'; in English we still speak of a depression as having 'lifted'.

It seems irrational, in the twenty-first century, to think of anorexia as a malignant enchantment, yet culturally it's the most plausible fit – a mood or conviction that brings misery and starvation, often arriving inexplicably and departing just as unaccountably. There may be warning signs: an unusual attitude to food before the illness came, a powerful determination to achieve goals, a destructive family dynamic, a traumatic experience, a perfectionist attention to detail, or any one of a number of other 'risk factors'. Each could have played a part in initiating an obsession with restricting food, but that doesn't explain why many people with odder attitudes to food, more destructive family dynamics, or greater perfectionism over details, never develop anorexia.

In some parts of the world shamans still use rituals to cast out malign spirits: as a family physician, in the modern West, anorexia can make me feel like a novice exorcist. Some of the anorexic patients I've known have succeeded, with or without help, to cast out the illness that was starving them; others found ways to make an uneasy truce with it. Some were defeated by their anorexia – it has the highest death rate of any mental illness. And it has been with us for centuries – St Catherine of Siena, who lived in the four-teenth century, was anorexic ('I pray to God and will pray, that He will grace me in this matter of eating so that I may live like other creatures'). So was the seventeenth-century nun Veronica Giuliani, a tortured woman who would lick walls and eat spiders, but not the meals placed before her in the convent refectory. It's not just a disorder of western culture: there are reports of anorexia from Nigeria, Hong Kong and South Africa, as well as among the Amish people (though one study from Fiji implied that television intro-duced anorexia to a community that had never known it).

Accounts from the Middle Ages, written by priests and abbesses charged with the care of anorexic nuns, betray feelings of bewilderment and impotence in the face of the illness that are comparable to those I've heard expressed by therapists in modern psychiatric clinics. Anorexia has been intimately, painfully and eloquently described by many men and women who have suffered it, and my perspective as a clinician is no substitute for those accounts.

SIMONE WAS A LAW STUDENT who hobbled into my office holding her stomach, complaining of overwhelming nausea and a light-headed sensation as if she was about to faint. I helped her onto the examination couch; the wings of her pelvic bones stretched the skin at her hips, and her ribs were a bowed washboard. Her abdomen was distended into a dome. 'It must be gas,' I thought to myself, 'maybe she's got a bowel obstruction.' But the swelling felt dull beneath my tapping finger, as if there was little air or gas beneath the skin. Her temperature was normal, and her blood pressure was on the low side for someone suffering so much pain. Most people with an obstruction in the bowel can't stop vomiting, but Simone didn't even retch. When the bowel is blocked by a twist or a tumour, the intestine works harder to clear the obstruction: intestinal fluids trickle through the interconnecting caverns of the bowel making high-pitched, tinkling sounds. But when I put a stethoscope on Simone's abdomen, it was silent.

'What have you had to eat in the last twenty-four hours?' I asked, gently pressing my hand over the quadrants of her swollen abdomen.

'Nothing unusual,' she said, grimacing. Her eyes looked trapped and frightened, like a stowaway under an opening hatch. 'A rice salad last night, and this morning a bit of toast.'

I slid a needle into her vein at the elbow, drew out a few tubes of blood for the lab, then gave her some anti-nausea medication and morphine. 'You're very dehydrated,' I told her, 'I'd like to arrange an ambulance to take you down to the hospital.' She lay back on the couch and nodded. White, downy hair on her cheeks, illuminated by the overhead strip lights, made a ragged, tilted corona around her face. 'Come and see me when you get out.'

It was a couple of weeks before she came back to see me, and her discharge letter held a surprise. 'Acute gastric dilatation with foodstuffs,' it said: 'Therapeutic Procedure: Decompression gastrotomy.' Simone had stitches down the front of her belly: the surgeons at the hospital had opened her up and found a stomach bulging with around six pints of half-chewed rice and melted ice cream. They'd piped it out with a tube, repaired the hole in her stomach, and stitched her up again.

The food restriction of anorexia leads to emaciation and malnutrition, while most men and women I've known with bulimia – whose eating disorder takes the form of self-induced vomiting or other purging – maintain a normal weight. But there's a grey zone between the two, variants of anorexia that are haunted by the compulsions of bulimia. In 'binge-purge anorexia', sufferers survive years of semi-starvation only to binge as a response to some stressor, sometimes as rarely as once every few years. A stomach shrivelled through disuse can't cope with the burden of a normal meal, so a binge stretches it perilously thin, and vomiting the foodstuffs out becomes impossible. It was clear that Simone had eaten so much food that her stomach, like her skin and bones, had been taken to breaking point.

I NEVER KNEW SIMONE'S PARENTS; on the couple of occasions I went to the home she shared with them, they weren't there. Over the months, then years, that I was Simone's doctor I found out more about her, and how anorexia nudged its way into her life. It took root like a spore in shadowed soil. She had always been slender and quiet, an only child, and the family was affluent: her mother was an academic who commuted between Edinburgh and Oxford, and her father a lawyer. They lived in a modern luxury apartment overlooking one of the city's parks, with sleek designer furniture and wide, echoing rooms.

Some anorexia begins in imitation – it's commoner among siblings of anorexic people and in pupils attending boarding schools – but in Simone's case it began with a fear of contamination. She picked up an infective diarrhoea – a common enough illness – that left her for a few weeks with cramping abdominal pain every time she ate. At first she thought that she was being recurrently infected by intestinal parasites, then that she was being poisoned by new food intolerances. She began to manipulate her diet to exclude potential triggers. Alone for much of the time in an empty flat with her textbooks, she commenced an obsessional hygiene routine, and began to categorise and weigh her food into 'good' and 'bad'. 'Bad food' insidiously became categorised in her mind as 'too fattening'. Most of us when we are hungry become distracted, irritable and light-headed, but Simone had a paradoxical reaction – she felt clean, clear-headed and calm. At first, her studies improved. She felt a new level of control over life and her circumstances.

Gradually, Simone's worries over being contaminated or

poisoned by food began to give way to a horror of the sated feeling that comes with a normal meal. She approached her meals distrustfully, pushing food around the plate as if engaged in bomb disposal rather than nourishment. In the early days, she'd stand in front of the refrigerator for a quarter of an hour, agonising over what to eat before walking away empty-handed. Later she avoided the refrigerator altogether. She took up running, experimenting with how little she could eat and still manage to complete her favourite circuit of the park without feeling faint. The circuit lengthened; the fat that all of us need for health, to cushion our bones, muscles and organs, began to melt from her hips, cheeks, shoulders. Her bones thinned, her ankles swelled with fluid from malnutrition, and she felt cold all the time. Her family life had never been particularly harmonious but mealtimes with her parents, frantic with concern about how to make her eat, became a battleground. It was after a particularly violent argument with them that she'd gorged on the rice and ice cream that had brought her to my clinic.

When we met again after the hospital admission I referred Simone urgently to the local eating disorders clinic. The psychiatrists recommended citalopram, an antidepressant medication which they hoped would help reduce some of her anxieties around eating, and they arranged fortnightly meetings both with themselves and with a dietician. 'They gave me sheets showing the minimum I have to eat to slowly bring up my weight,' Simone told me at one of the early appointments. 'I'm sticking to them, I really am.' But her weight didn't rise. Deception is an inextricable part of most eating disorders, and I found out later that she never took the citalopram as prescribed, and rarely ate as the dieticians advised. Her periods had stopped long before, but now her ankle swelling worsened, and downy hair grew even more thickly on her cheeks.* She dropped out of law school.

---

* The downy hair growth is due to hormone imbalance. This 'lanugo'

WHAT IS IT THAT CAUSES a healthy adolescent, whether male or female, to starve themselves until their bones soften, their teeth loosen, their hair falls out and their hearts weaken? Among the first to define it was a French physician, Charles Lasègue, who in 1873 gave a fairly sweeping summary of some of the characteristics he associated with the illness:

> A young girl, between fifteen and twenty years of age, suffers from some emotion which she avows or conceals. Generally it relates to some real or imaginary marriage project, to a violence done to some sympathy, or to some more or less conscient desire. At other times, only conjectures can be offered concerning the occasional cause.

As to ideas about causes, the same could be said today: 'only conjectures can be offered'. As a constellation of attitudes to food and body weight, anorexia transcends times and beliefs, but its triggers involve a pernicious synergy of culture, advertising, peer pressure, genetics, family relationships, storms of hormones and peculiarities of personality. It's often precipitated by some stressful life event: a bereavement, challenge or change in role.

The journalist Katy Waldman, a recovered anorexic, wrote an eloquent, fearless essay about her illness which noted some of the contradictions at its heart. She pointed out that there's a tendency among survivors to make a poetry of emaciation: anorexia becomes a choreographed performance that ultimately becomes a prison. She called for an end to the celebration of wan, delicate women in art and literature, and a rejection of destructive narratives that seek to amplify their appeal. The illness awakens a revulsion towards food and a healthy body weight that seems unassailable, perhaps because it is so closely associated with the

---

or 'wool-like' hair has led some scholars to speculate that the medieval nuns canonised as 'bearded saints' suffered from anorexia.

primitive aspects of our humanity: nourishment, sexuality, body awareness. For adolescents, it provokes a retrogression of puberty, seeming at first to effect a transformation in reverse. 'I starved,' wrote Waldman, 'to acquire that old classical capability: metamorphosis.'

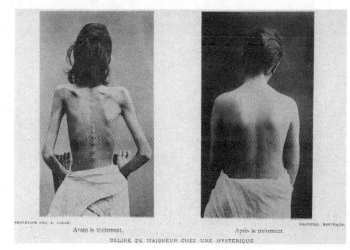

Avant le traitement.   Après le traitement.

DÉLIRE DE MAIGREUR CHEZ UNE HYSTÉRIQUE

If anorexia is, as Waldman proposes, a kind of dramatic performance, Simone and I tried to sneak in new stage directions. I wanted to exploit her formidable perfectionism and resolve to an alternative end: a healthy weight. We agreed together a list of foods she'd endeavour to eat at breakfast, lunch and dinner, tabulating their associated calories – she accepted that without a minimum intake her body would grow weaker, and her mind too. But none of my interventions seemed to hold; her revulsion at the feeling of a modest meal within her stomach remained strong, and her weight continued to fluctuate on the edge of what is compatible with life. Twice more she was admitted to hospital: once when the salt levels in her blood threatened to destabilise the rhythms of her heart, and once when she collapsed unconscious with low blood pressure. I asked her once, 'Do you think there's a part of you that would welcome death?', and she took a long time in answering.

But the answer, when it came, was 'no', and after three years of our meetings, her breakthrough came. I can't take any credit for the change: after numerous medications, dieticians, admissions to hospital and regular visits to the psychiatrists, one day she told me simply that she'd eaten a chocolate bar, and felt better. 'It was that simple,' she said, astonished by the obviousness of what she needed to do. 'I had energy. I felt good. I was expecting that horrid feeling to come over me, that disgust, but it didn't. And I had only the one – I didn't gorge on them.'

'What made the difference?' I asked her.

'No idea – it's just that now when I feel nauseated at the idea of eating, I can see it as a sign that I'm not thinking straight, a sign that I actually *have to* eat.'

Over the subsequent months I charted the rise of Simone's weight back into health. She returned to law school, moved out of her parents' flat, started dating, and though she never lost her perfectionism, her dedicated attention to the ingredients of what she ate, her weight didn't drop the way it had over those three years.

Much later, when the downy hair had gone from her cheeks, she had strength in her limbs and the rhythms of her hormones had returned, she came to see me about contraceptive pills. 'Remember those awful years,' she said and gave a short laugh, 'the only good thing about them was that my periods stopped.'

'Do you ever think about those years now?' I asked her.

'Sometimes,' she replied. 'It's hazy though, as if I was under a spell. I wish I knew how it was broken.'

11

Hallucination: A Sphere of Devils

For man has closed himself up, till he sees all things through narrow chinks of his cavern.

William Blake, *The Marriage of Heaven and Hell*

I HAVE A PATIENT who believes her fingers are rotting. Usually Megan offers me her fingertips for inspection. Her unclipped nails are thick with grime, and more than once I've led her to the sink where together we've scrubbed them with a nail brush. 'Can't you smell it?' she asks me, 'they're disgusting.' I don't smell or see anything unusual. Megan is sometimes tormented by bullying and insulting voices, and when those voices are strong, so are the hallucinations of rot. We meet at least once a month: for me, it's a chance to check how she's getting on; for her, it's to pick up her antipsychotic drug prescription. She finds the drugs helpful; the consultations, I think, less so. I've tried exploring what the rotten fingertips might mean for her; whether they're a symbol of some rot or canker that gnaws at her mind rather than her fingers. 'Nope, there's nothing symbolic about it,' she says. 'They *really* stink. I can't believe you can't smell it.'

In Greek the word 'psyche' means 'soul' or 'life'; 'psychosis' means 'animation' or 'infusing with life'. For nineteenth- and early twentieth-century psychiatrists it meant something different: 'psychosis' was madness arising from a disorder of mind, as opposed to 'neurosis', which arose from a disorder of nerves (this is now recognised to be a meaningless distinction). Today the word is reserved for those who hold beliefs and report hallucinatory perceptions that are manifestly untrue – those who've lost touch in a particularly damaging or distressing way with what's verifiably real. In *Dementia Praecox, or the Group of Schizophrenias*, published in 1911, psychiatrist Eugen Bleuler coined the term 'schizophrenia' to describe a group of mental illnesses that suggested this loss of grip on reality. His book affirmed that when delusions or hallucinations become prominent, 'everything may seem different; one's own person as well as the external world ... The person loses his boundaries in time and space.' In schizophrenia, this loss of boundaries can become enduring, life-limiting and profoundly distressing.

When people take hallucinogenic drugs for pleasure, that pleasure is contingent on the change they offer being temporary. Aldous Huxley's *Doors of Perception*, an essay exploring the effects of taking four-tenths of a gramme of the hallucinogenic drug mescaline, took its title from William Blake: 'If the doors of perception were cleansed, every thing would appear to man as it is, infinite.' For Huxley, the brain was a reducing valve, optimised to restrict the glory and plurality of the world. He took hallucinogens with the intention of blowing open that valve, and specifically noted that the drug gave him an 'inkling' of what it might feel like to be psychotic. He wanted to induce a transformed state of consciousness, and shortcut through to the ecstatic states of mystical religion like those described by practitioners of Zen Buddhism, in which perceptual boundaries are said to be similarly dissolved.

The idea that drugs could offer transcendence was criticised by the Zen master D. T. Suzuki, who insisted that hallucinogenic drugs gave an insight only into a 'devil's sphere' of reality. Taking LSD, Suzuki is quoted as saying, 'is stupid'. 'These drugs conjure up "mystic" visions,' he wrote, '[but] Zen is concerned not with these visions, as the drug-takers are, but with the "person" who is the subject of the visions.' Suzuki's student Koji Sato took a different view: hallucinogenic drugs gave access to a mental state in which students 'should not linger', but from which much could be learned. Sato tells the story of one Zen student who couldn't progress beyond a series of Buddhist koan teachings until he took LSD; following his drug experiences, he 'passed these koans easily'.

It seems a universal that human minds seek to move in and out of alternative worlds, altering their state of consciousness. Children accomplish these transformations through play, but with adults, drugs are an almost ubiquitous feature of human communities, whether to transform perspective, become energised or to relax. Almost every society has a tradition of using drugs, and the few without tend to have developed alternative means of accessing hallucinatory states such as fasting, or prolonged meditation.

Broadly speaking, to be an hallucinogen, a drug must induce a distortion of perception without acting as a sedative or stimulant. There are many natural hallucinogens, and their use by humans has been described as far back as the Hindu Vedas – about 5,000 years. In the Middle Ages there were periodic outbreaks of a condition known as St Anthony's Fire, in which whole communities experienced hallucinations when they ate bread contaminated with ergot alkaloids. The alkaloids are generated by a fungus that grows on grain; in the gut they cause diarrhoea and vomiting, and in the brain they can cause headaches, hallucinations and seizures. A similar effect is brought on by ingesting the leaves or berries of deadly nightshade ('belladonna'). One seventeenth-century treatise on belladonna poisoning emphasised the religious and mystical nature of the hallucinations – prefiguring Huxley's *Doors of Perception.*

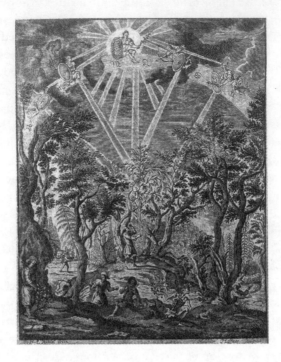

There are many other natural drugs that have hallucinogenic effects, like the psilocybin of mushrooms, and the peyote of Meso-American cacti. But the most powerful hallucinogen of all is a synthetic one, Lysergic acid, or LSD. It's active in tiny doses, about a thousandth of the equivalent dose of mescaline, making it one of the most powerful drugs known: 10μg can produce a feeling of euphoria, and as little as 50μg an hallucinogenic effect.

LSD was first synthesised in 1938, but its effect wasn't discovered until 1943 when, while working in the laboratory, the Swiss chemist Albert Hoffman accidentally absorbed some through his fingers. He thought he had died and been transported to hell. The drug has wide-ranging effects across the brain, and scientists couldn't figure out how it transformed vision, hearing, smelling and dreaming without dulling or heightening the taker's level of consciousness. In the 1950s and 1960s it was trialled as a therapy for alcoholism, for depression, even for schizophrenia, but few studies have been able to prove any enduring therapeutic benefit. More recently, the psilocybin of hallucinogenic mushrooms has been proposed as an aid to deepen engagement in psychotherapy, much as Sato's Zen student passed the most difficult koans only after taking hallucinogens. But LSD is not without danger: many studies show a small, persistent risk of psychotic reactions to the drug – around 1 or 2 per cent. It seems that LSD-induced visions can cede to hallucinatory states that persist long after the drug itself has been eliminated from the body.

MY INTRODUCTION AS A MEDICAL STUDENT to the horror of drug-induced psychosis was Dan, a young student of philosophy I met during a psychiatry attachment. After taking LSD for the first time, Dan had a psychotic reaction with persistent hallucinations, and disabling panic attacks. I spent a couple of hours talking with him about his experience. He was short, with blonde curls to each side of his forehead like question marks, and a vertical line between his eyebrows like an exclamation. Angry patches of acne erupted between the sparse bristles on his cheeks.

He told me that he took a tab of the drug one evening in his bedroom, out of curiosity. The first thing he noticed, within twenty minutes or so, was that his bed was breathing, the quilt was rising and falling in time with his own breath. He tried to write down 'the bed is breathing' on a piece of paper, but the sensation of the pen on paper was all wrong, as if the nib was sinking through into the wooden desk beneath. Lying down on his bed he glanced up out of the window, and noticed that the sky was pulsing between light and dark. 'It wasn't frightening at first,' he said, 'but beautiful'; he lay for a while mesmerised by the change. He knocked on his flatmate's door to tell him about the vision but found that instead of words, only giggles would come out. 'Every time I tried to speak it was as if I had to line the words up beforehand in some antechamber of my mind,' he said, 'then blurt them out. But they wouldn't come.' On a trip to the toilet he saw his urine as fluorescent green blobs on the porcelain, beautifully bright, like scales on a dragon-fly. As he watched, they seemed to spiral in a vortex towards the base of the pan before melting away.

At first the drug made him feel exhilarated and euphoric: he wanted to go out and enjoy his new perceptions. He strode out for a walk around the neighbourhood, but the euphoria quickly melted: his feet on the pavement seemed to sink into the cement; the music playing through his ear-phones began to boom from the brick walls of the buildings around him. His exhilaration yielded to a creeping, desolat-ing anxiety. Beneath the hood of a pedestrian he glimpsed the flashing impression of a skull. Every piece of chewing gum trodden into the pavement glowed red, green or amber depending on the light showing at its nearest traffic lights. A panic attack came over him, bringing a toxic paranoia: every car looked like a police car, every pedestrian seemed like a threat.

He cut the walk short and, running back to his flat, noticed that the drug had done something to his body tem-perature – he was overheating. Once back in his room he stripped off all his clothes, and sat naked in the middle of the bedroom. 'I kept telling myself, "What can happen to you? You're here, on your bedroom floor, nothing bad can happen"'. But a great deal was happening: the edges of the posters on his walls were moving, scraps of paint on the wooden floor seemed to writhe like larvae, and when he looked down at his skin, it seemed to swirl in endless migra-tion over its own surface. 'It was terrifying to see that even my body wasn't safe,' he said. 'But it was also horribly fascinating: my hand would transform between looking old, wrinkled and weak, then it'd become strong, youthful and powerful. And if I looked in the mirror I'd see the same rapid change, backwards and forwards, on my face.'

Dan sat for hours like that on his bedroom floor, too scared to switch off the lights and sleep, terrified to leave the room. 'I felt as if I'd passed my whole life perched on a plinth in a central chamber of my mind,' he said. 'Stable and secure. That night I was kicked off, and left hanging by my fingernails over some awful chasm. I knew that if I let go, I'd go mad.'

By sunrise the following day he was still flinching at unexpected auditory hallucinations, distrustful of every sensation – even the hard pressure of the floor beneath him. Music would blare loud then become muted, and he flinched at flickering shadows on the edges of his vision. Sleepless now for thirty hours, his paranoia was intensified by exhaustion: he became overwhelmed by terror at the prospect of going outside. His flatmate called the GP, and then accompanied him to the local clinic. The GP sent him in a taxi to the emergency psychiatric team at the local hospital, where he sweated, trembled and stared at the floor until he was seen.

'They told me it would fade with time and they were right,' Dan said. 'They gave me some drugs – sedatives – that brought such relief. The first one I took was like honey on my brain.' The psychiatric team arranged to see him again the following day – he didn't need to be admitted into the hospital ward. The new drug slowed him down, his thoughts became viscous, and he had to stop attending the university. But within three weeks he had reduced the dose to a negligible amount, and was learning to breathe through the panic attacks. Out on the street he still saw skulls on people's faces, but was finding ways of ignoring the visions and distracting himself. Speaking to medical students like me was one of the ways in which he was trying to understand his experience, and reclaim his mind.

THE PSYCHIATRIST R. D. LAING spent many hundreds of hours listening to personal accounts of psychosis. There are striking similarities between his case reports and accounts like Dan's of a terrifying LSD trip. In *The Divided Self* Laing quotes one of his psychotic patients: 'I'm losing myself. It's getting deeper and deeper. I want to tell you things, but I'm scared.' In his book *Disembodied Spirits and Deanimated Bodies*, Italian psychiatrist Giovanni Stanghellini quotes a patient undergoing a similar kind of 'ego disintegration': 'All sensations seem to be different from usual and to fall apart. My body is changing, my face too. I feel disconnected from myself.'

There's a theory about schizophrenia that proposes psychosis as a disintegration of the moment-to-moment synthesis between the different social and mental roles we inhabit – a synthesis we all carry out unconsciously, and which hallucinogens temporarily disrupt. From this perspective, psychosis and hallucinogenic drugs break the tiller that allows us to navigate between inner and outer worlds. Each of us is composed of bundles of different identities, and we are subject to ceaseless torrents of sensory awareness; in psychosis the ability to create wholeness from that turmoil breaks down. Images from functional MRI scanners are notoriously difficult to interpret and the technology is still in its infancy, but when the brains of LSD users are visualised, networks of neurons that under normal circumstances all fire together can be seen to become desynchronised. It may be an insight into how those many selves that constitute our being can be shattered apart.

Dan found a way back from the edge of disintegration and his breakdown, though provoked by a drug, gave me a glimpse of what some of my patients with schizophrenia, like Megan, might be going through. Hallucinogens can offer visions but risk division of the self, and for Albert Hoffman, Dan, and for D. T. Suzuki, those visions are a 'sphere of devils'. But for many users the effects are pleasing, compelling, addictive, even heavenly. Precisely because they are temporary, they offer some an escape when life feels tedious, and bring breadth and richness when it feels narrow or impoverished. But it's a fragile heaven they offer: dissolving the boundaries of experience may become a dark hell of terror. To reassert the boundaries of perception is to offer a path back to the light.

12

Puberty: Suddenly Accelerated Youth

With man the young arrive at maturity at a much later age than with any other animal.

Charles Darwin, *The Descent of Man*

I WORKED ONCE with a wise and straight-talking community midwife, a mother of four, who after delivering babies at home would visit regularly for the first few days to check how well couples were adapting to becoming parents. I asked if there were any impressions or insights she'd gathered over the decades of her work. Some take a first baby in their stride, she told me, while others felt as if parenthood had dropped them into a tunnel of fear and exhaustion. It often seemed to her as if the younger the parents, the less difficulty they had adapting to the change.

'Do you give them any advice?' I asked her.

'The ones who are struggling? I tell them that for the first six or seven years kids just need you,' she replied, 'and you have to find a way of reconciling yourself to that. But then the following six or seven are just lovely, as the children learn about the world, and get slowly more independent.'

'And the six or seven years after that?' I asked.

'They go somewhere you can't follow,' she said and gave a wistful smile. 'But mostly they come back.'

In clinic I see plenty of babies, toddlers and pre-school children – often with wheezes, fevers, ear infections and rashes. Sometimes there are concerns about feeding, and sometimes about growth. By about the age of six the frequency of visits drops away, as the kids get better at fighting off infections, and hit their stride in terms of development. But then at age twelve or thirteen I start to see them again, as the hormonal upheavals of adolescence take hold.

All babies produce sex hormones: I often see unweaned newborns of both sexes with swollen breast tissue created by oestrogen. But the brain of a newborn baby is trigger-sensitive to sex hormones, and a sensitive feedback mechanism, initiated soon after birth, slams a brake on their production. The sensitivity of that brake diminishes in late childhood until it's weak enough, finally, to activate puberty. The onset of puberty isn't then the unfolding of something new, but a release into something that's been long suppressed.

There's a famous painting by Edvard Munch, created during his anxious years in Berlin, which shows a naked pubescent girl with flushed cheeks and a defiant, quizzical gaze. He called it simply *Pubertet* – 'puberty'. She's sitting on the edge of a bed, wrists crossed in her lap, hair loose over the shoulders. The most striking aspect of the image is not the boldness of her stare, or the finesse with which she's been painted, but a large, womb-shaped shadow that bulges up from beneath her onto the wall.

Some critics reckon that the shadow represents Munch's own repressed sexuality; others think it's a phallic symbol or symbol of the womb, or that it represents the challenges and complexities of looming adult life. Many parents welcome the gathering strength and independence they see in their children, while others mourn the arrival of puberty as a loss of innocence. Munch's painting implies that the coming of sexual maturity is a kind of expulsion from the Eden of childhood into the solitude and the responsibilities of adult life.

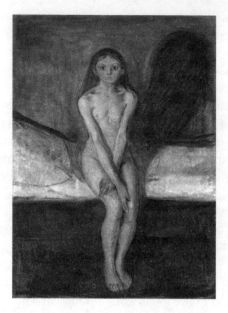

I MET BILLIE BAXTER when she was four years old, when two long-term patients of my practice adopted her. She was small for her age, inquisitive and agile, with short blonde hair that curled at the nape of the neck. As soon as she entered my office she'd make straight for a mat of toys, then jump on the weighing scales. Her mother Amy worked as a librarian, and her father Simon stayed home to look after Billie.

Ear infections, chest infections, constipation, eczema – over the first couple of years I saw a fair amount of Billie. She stayed small for her age. If you measure the heights and weights of one hundred children, and plot them on charts, it's usual to show the 'normal' range as existing between the third-smallest and the third-largest child: the '3rd centile' and the '97th centile' respectively. Billie stayed around the 5th centile, at the lower end of the normal range. Billie's inquisitiveness remained with her – she was bright at nursery, and once at school proved to be a precocious reader. Little was known about her birth parents.

I never had to visit Simon and Amy at home, and by the time Billie was six the frequency of her visits to the clinic dropped away. A year after I'd last seen her I received a questionnaire from a life insurance company for Amy. I rang up to see how they were all getting on: Simon told me that the infections had stopped bothering Billie, her eczema had settled down, and that she was no longer troubled with constipation.

A couple of years later, when Billie was eight, I saw her name on my clinic list again. She sat in the chair by my desk, swinging her legs and looking around as if remembering all those childhood visits. She was wearing unicorn-patterned trousers and a sweater printed with a kitten – her hair had darkened with age and she held it back in a ponytail. She looked about average size for her age – she must have been approaching the 50th centile. 'I've come to ask you about her toes,' said Amy, 'the nails are growing in at the corners.' Billie took off her trainers – she had glitter varnish on every toenail – and I showed her how to lift up the corners with pieces of cotton wool so they wouldn't dig into the flesh. When I'd finished, and Billie had put her socks and trainers back on, Amy asked her to go and wait outside.

'I wanted to speak to you on your own,' Amy said as soon as the door was closed. 'When is it normal to start puberty?'

'Well, that depends …' I began.

'Because I was twelve before my periods started,' Amy went on.

'Has Billie had a period?'

'No, not a period, but her breasts are starting to grow. She's only eight!'

'Has she any pubic hair yet?' I asked her.

She shook her head. 'No, thank goodness. It couldn't be starting already, could it?'

THE SEQUENCE AND TIMING of puberty was first worked out in the 1960s by James Tanner, a paediatrician at the Institute of Child Health in London, and his colleague W. A. Marshall. As a medical student I had to memorise the sequence, so as to be able to recognise when it went awry. No periods in a girl with mature bones suggested an underlying gynaecological problem; pubic hair before breast or testicle growth suggested a hormonal problem, and so on.

My textbook in paediatrics carried cartoon drawings based on Tanner and Marshall's seminal papers, showing the progressive changes in boys' genitalia, girls' breasts and both sexes' pubic hair, alongside normal age ranges for each stage. According to Tanner, the photographs the cartoons were based on were taken at an orphanage called the Harpenden Children's Home just north of London – the focus of a study that had examined the growth of children since 1951. For two days every month throughout the period of the study one of Tanner's colleagues, R. H. Whitehouse, visited the children's home. Whitehouse took naked photographs of the boys and girls one at a time, making sure they were timed to capture images within fifteen days of their birthdays. In total each child was photographed twice yearly in childhood, and four times yearly as adolescents, because the rate of change in adolescence is so much greater; 192 girls and 228 boys took part.

It's not clear from Tanner's research publications how much choice the children had about taking part. It must have been an unsettling sight: scores of children queuing nervously for a room in which each had to strip for a photographer. Whitehouse worked 'at a rate of three or four per hour'. The photographs were taken as frontal and profile images, collated by name, and later assessed by Tanner and Marshall. 'The development of the secondary sex characters was studied in whole-body photographs,' wrote Tanner, 'By comparing each picture with the preceding one, changes in the genitalia and pubic hair could be readily recognized.'

But the images they gathered have been fundamental to the understanding of the way puberty evolves, and the medical understanding of how to intervene when it goes wrong. The two men classified pubertal development into five discrete stages, and created tables to facilitate the staging of development for the clinician. In the profile photographs each child was arranged to face their younger selves, as if looking back with longing towards their own childhood.

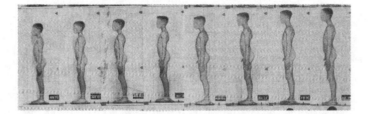

Arranged in sequence, the photographs stood as a cinematography of the transformations of puberty.

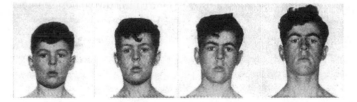

In the materials and methods section of their paper, Tanner and Marshall described all the participants as 'white British' and that 'they had no physical abnormalities, and lived in small family groups in a children's home where the standard of care was in all respects excellent'. Online, there are plenty of testimonies agreeing that Harpenden was an excellent institution, though you don't have to look far to find poignant tales of unhappiness, as well as furious allegations of abuse. Socio-economically it was a skewed population; Tanner admitted that the children 'came mainly from the lower socio-economic sector of the population, and some may not have received optimal physical care before entering the home (usually between age 3 and 6 years)'.

Being neglected as a child, and being of low birth weight, has been found in some studies to bring puberty forward through a mechanism that remains unknown, as if the human evolutionary response to a stressful childhood is to facilitate pregnancy in the next generation as quickly as possible. This process is known as 'early life programming'; Tanner's children may have entered puberty earlier than the average through this mechanism, and so weren't representative of the general population. It's well recognised that children like those at Harpenden who begin life in a resource-poor environment but move to be brought up in a resource-rich environment, go into puberty earlier than the natives of either environment that stayed put. The same process happens in plants – those that begin in poor soil, and are then given richer soil, reproduce earlier and more abundantly. At the same time the *average* age of menarche or menophany – the age when girls first have a period – has dropped overall in the United States and in western Europe from around age seventeen in the mid-nineteenth century to age thirteen by the mid-twentieth, for reasons that are still unclear.*

---

* In 1939 a Peruvian girl called Lina Medina became the youngest recorded mother, giving birth by caesarean section to a baby boy at the age of five years and eight months. Lina reportedly began menstruating

BILLIE WAS YOUNG to show the earliest signs of puberty, but according to Tanner's charts her development was within the normal range – just as she was in the lowest centiles for height, she was in the lowest centiles for pubertal onset: the second, visible stage of breast development can be reached as early as eight and a half. Perhaps her life before adoption had influenced her early puberty, or perhaps her own birth mother had been the same.

It was a couple of years before I saw Billie in my office again – Amy told me before the appointment that she'd been teased at school for wearing a bra, and her first period had come just before her tenth birthday. She was now among the tallest in the class. She sat in the chair by my desk, big for her age, wearing dark, baggy jeans and a black hooded sweatshirt. She no longer swung her legs or looked interestedly around the room, but held her hands in the front pocket of the sweatshirt, her shoulders hunched forwards.

'The first thing is her acne,' said Amy; 'you can see it on her forehead, and she's getting it on her shoulders too.' The skin was shiny and speckled with little pustules. Billie sank even further, if it was possible, into her chair.

'I can help with that,' I told her, and lightly tugged back the hood on the sweatshirt to have a closer look. 'I'll give you some lotions and if it's no better within a couple of months let me know – there's other things we can do.' A glance of relief shot across Billie's face, like sunlight between clouds, but she still didn't say anything.

'And then there's her knees – she gets these terrible pains when she runs, or after sports in school,' Amy said. 'And they've got lumps on them too. Come on, Billie,' she added with a hint of impatience, 'show Dr Francis.'

Billie gave a sigh, and rolled up her jeans to show me

---

at around a year old. Edmundo Escomel, 'La plus jeune mère du monde', *La Presse Médicale* vol. 47, no. 43, 1939, p. 875.

her knees; she had hard, tender swellings on her shins just below the kneecaps.

'That's just because you're growing so quickly just now,' I said. 'You can think of it as your bones growing faster than your tendons.' I pulled over the skeleton that stands in my clinic room, and pointed out where the tendon from the kneecap attaches to the shin, and how its traction could pull up and irritate the bone. 'It's even got a name, this condition,' I added, 'Osgood-Schlatter's disease.' Billie snorted a laugh.

The growth rate of bones after babyhood through childhood is fairly constant, but the sex hormones of puberty accelerate that background rate. Tanner and Marshall showed that graphs of 'height velocity' throughout childhood take the shape of a ski jump, because the rapid growth of babyhood falls away only to shoot up again in early adolescence. Tanner and Marshall's papers are a model of dispassionate clinical language, but occasionally a note of humanity breaks through, showing that they were concerned not only with their research, but with the anxieties that all teenagers feel around puberty: 'All the girls in this study … had passed the peak of their height spurt before menstruation began,' they wrote; 'We can therefore confidently reassure the tall girl who has reached menarche at an early age that her growth is now slowing down.' Tanner also acknowledged the institutionalised sexism of the 1950s with reference to a paper from the American psychologist L. K. Frank: 'adolescence, at least in urban American girls, is a period of considerable stress and perplexity; [Frank] lays particular emphasis on the difficulty these girls find in accepting with satisfaction the feminine role.'

SEX HORMONES AFFECT the male breasts too – it's not uncommon to have to reassure adolescent boys whose nipples are swollen and tender that they aren't turning into girls. With time their symptoms almost always settle down. The first sign of puberty in boys is a loosening of their scrotum, giving way to an increase in the size of their testicles, and the first pubic hair. The enlarging testicles make more and more testosterone, which in turn drives other changes: an increase in the size of the penis, a darkening of the scrotal skin.

Pubic hair growth is driven not so much by testosterone, but by steroid hormones produced in the adrenal glands – that's why it occurs in girls as much as it does in boys. Those same hormones also drive a change in the sweat glands: so-called 'apocrine' glands become active, which make oilier, smellier secretions than the more watery sweat glands active in childhood (as anyone who has ever washed a teenager's socks will confirm). The same hormones bring an increased tendency for pores on the face, chest and shoulders to get plugged and infected, provoking eruptions of acne. In both sexes the larynx lengthens and broadens, deepening the voice, but in boys this deepening effect becomes more pronounced.

And the transformations of puberty entail more than just the visible: there are substantial changes in the brain. An increase in risk-taking behaviour and aggression in boys has been tentatively correlated to a delay in maturation of the pre-frontal areas of the cortex. It's thought that our capacities for abstract reasoning, and perception of social cues, go on improving into our twenties. For reasons that aren't quite clear, teenage brains recalibrate to a different, later, body clock: for the average teenager, 7 a.m. feels the same way for them as 5 a.m. does for someone middle-aged. In 1955 Tanner caricatured the folk wisdom about adolescence:

> A picture is painted of the suddenly accelerated youth, staggering under the impact of his newly acquired hormones … Mutually incompatible drives and emotions are simultaneously aroused, many of which later become shed or repressed bit by bit as the individual chooses inevitably this path rather than that.

Or as the midwife I once worked with told me, they go somewhere you can't follow, but then they come back.

Many adolescents develop anxieties around body image that are intimately connected to the rapid transformations of their bodies. Tempestuous shifts in mood through adolescence are found across cultures, irrespective of wealth (though one study in the United States found that African Americans were uniquely protected against body image anxieties, for obscure reasons). Puberty can entail intense psychosocial upheaval, of questioning the choices and the wisdom of the adults around us – it becomes a fire through which some aspects of our childhood selves are burned away, while others are annealed into elements of our adult identity.

The final act in the drama of puberty is the closure of the growth plates of bone, the timing of which is the same across human populations irrespective of ethnicity. Epiphyses fuse in a particular order – understanding the correct sequence is essential when reviewing X-rays in the emergency department so that, as a doctor, you can distinguish between a flake of bone chipped off through an injury, or a healthy flake of bone that has simply yet to fuse. Long bones, such as the femur or the humerus, may not fully fuse until age twenty-one, and in women, the pelvis may grow until as late as twenty-two.

When Charles Darwin began to think about puberty, he noticed how striking the delay in human puberty, in comparison with other primates. Human babies have the largest heads relative to the body size of any mammals, and without that late, broadening growth of the pelvis in young women, babies would struggle to be born. But it can't be just about the skeleton: in the timing and the traumas of human adolescence, there's some recognition that human nature and society is complex, and it takes us years to figure out how to position ourselves as part of the adult world.

13

Pregnancy: The Most Meticulous Work

'Good God!' says he, 'how snug and compleat it lies – I defy all our painters in St Martins lane to put a Child into such a situation.'

William Hogarth, on seeing the dissection of a foetus *in utero*

ULTRASOUND SCANS were first developed in Glasgow, by a professor of midwifery called Ian Donald who had heard of metalworkers using them to detect flaws in steel. The metalworkers would calibrate the ultrasound machines against their thumbs, because bone and flesh reflect sound waves differently. In the summer of 1955, Donald drove from Glasgow down to a boiler manufacturers in Renfrew, his car boot full of buckets of ovarian cysts and uterine tumours. He compared ultrasound images of the body parts with those he obtained from a slab of steak. Impressed with the results, he moved the machine out of the metallurgists' workshop and into the clinic.

In 1958 he wrote up his findings in a paper called 'The Investigation of Abdominal Masses by Pulsed Ultrasound.' The sound waves worked as well to outline the dimensions of a baby's skull as they did a cyst or a tumour, and Donald began refining the technique to monitor the growth and development of babies in the womb. Within a couple of decades his scanners were ubiquitous: I've seen cheap and simple machines used upcountry in East and West Africa, and in rural clinics in India. They're indispensable now for monitoring the growth and development of the baby, to identify the position of the placenta (if it is too near the cervix it risks rupture in labour). They're even used in the frenzy of delivery itself for a quick check of the baby's precise position.

The technology has moved on: it's possible these days to watch babies on ultrasound in three dimensions. The internet is suffused with these images; often the sonogram image is shown side by side with a photograph of the same baby hours after birth. Mothers bring printouts to my clinic: asteroidal contours pixelate against a black, starless background, reminiscent of images beamed back from deep space. But a closer inspection reveals them to be the most human of forms, beamed not from the reaches of the solar system but from the future.

Perhaps it's the glimpse of the future they grant that makes these images so enchanting, or perhaps it's because through most of human history the transformations of pregnancy have been hidden. There's something transgressive, even uncanny, about them. Though woven by sound, they offer silent promises of what is to come.

AS A JUNIOR DOCTOR working in obstetrics I'd be asked to help out in antenatal clinics: a dozen or so women, in various stages of pregnancy, seen across the span of a morning. There was an ultrasound scanner somewhere behind a curtain but it wasn't for routine use – it was enough to use faster more traditional methods of determining whether a pregnancy was proceeding well. The checks I was to perform have been standardised across the world, and are so formulaic that each woman brought a list of them to each appointment on a grid. Date of clinic visit was written on the vertical axis, and each check was given a box to be ticked along a horizontal. To complete an antenatal check, it was enough to work your way across the grid.

Pregnant women have an increased blood volume, their hearts beating for two (or three, in the case of twins), which may drive blood pressure up. Their pulse rate too can accelerate to cope, and a particularly elevated pulse hints at a problem. Kidneys can be affected, and I'd dip-test a bottle of urine to make sure that there was no blood or protein leaking out. I'd draw a blood sample from each patient to see if the haemoglobin and platelets were keeping up with the extraordinary demands being made on them: the blood counts of most women drop during pregnancy, their blood diluted by the increased volume. And I'd ask them whether they were suffering from any of the customary complaints of pregnancy: nausea, backache, heartburn, or the bony pain of a stretching pelvis.

These checks were to gauge how much the effort of pregnancy was proving a strain on each woman's body; when they were complete I'd move on to check how the baby, or babies, were growing and changing in the womb. That new life may take root and, like some kind of magical fruit, begin to swell, is the most quotidian of marvels. But it *is* marvellous. It felt like a great privilege to chart that burgeoning change.

First to be assessed was the baby's 'lie' in the womb, trying to feel the weighty, solid roundness of a head, the curve of a spine, the smaller, softer and more mobile globe of a tiny rump. The further on the pregnancy the more significant the 'lie'; if the head was up ('breech'), a discussion would be opened with the midwives about whether to plan a caesarean or a vaginal delivery. Next I'd measure the 'height' of the womb itself, using nothing more advanced than a tape measure. Beyond the middle weeks of pregnancy, irrespective of size or ethnicity, the distance in centimetres, from the pubic bone to the uppermost extent of the womb correlates almost exactly to the number of weeks a woman has been pregnant. This correlation is so responsive that in the final weeks of pregnancy, when the baby's head drops deeper into the pelvis in preparation for labour I'd see a corresponding drop in this 'fundal height'.

In her elegant account of her own pregnancy, *Expecting*, Chitra Ramaswamy wrote of how comforting this element of the antenatal visit was for her:

> How reassuring to feel the old-school pressure of its end against the top of my pubic bone, drawing me up as if I were a length of fabric. Pregnancy was meticulous work, as precise as a dress pattern, and my bump always measured within a centimetre or so of the number of weeks I was pregnant.

The unravelled tape measure would follow the *linea nigra* or 'black line' of pregnancy, in which the skin from pubis to umbilicus darkens with the hormones of pregnancy. 'It bisected my stomach like a ring around a planet or a veined streak of quartz encircling a pebble,' wrote Ramaswamy, 'evidence of a disturbance within. Some mysterious ancient change.'

The final phase of the antenatal check, listening to the baby's heartbeat, was to be signed off on the grid with a scribbled 'FHH' – 'foetal heart heard' – a peremptory way to document something so auspicious. If foetal ultrasound images seem beamed from the future, so did these peculiar, mesmerising sounds: rapid, pristine heartbeats clattering above the stately bass of the mother's own pulse.

AFTER BILLIE BAXTER'S precocious puberty I didn't see her again until she was thirteen – having finished developing at an age when some boys have barely started. Amy brought her in. 'Billie's pregnant,' she said bluntly, as soon as they'd sat down, her face haloed in anger. 'I don't know how it happened, and she's certainly not telling.' Billie sat hunched in the chair by my desk, face hooded, arms folded, gaze fixed on the floor. She didn't know it, but she was mirroring her mum's posture. 'It doesn't matter who he is,' Billie said. 'I'm not seeing him any more. You can't make me get rid of it.'

'Who's going to look after the baby?' Amy said, her voice beseeching, then menacing. 'You can't drop out of school at fourteen. For God's sake, Billie!' She looked across at me, pleading now. 'I can't be a grandmother! Not yet!' Billie just folded her arms all the tighter. Her ex-boyfriend was fourteen, she said. She'd wanted to have sex with him. And she was going to have the baby.

In my area there are counsellors trained to support young women who've become pregnant in their teens, or need confidential advice about contraception. I picked up the phone and spoke to one of them – she gave me a time for Billie to attend the following day. I wrote the time and place on a slip of paper and handed it over, along with a prescription for some folic acid supplements. 'If you're sure you want to go ahead with this pregnancy, take one of these each day,' I said, 'they're good for the baby.' She sighed, took the prescription and stuffed it into her pocket.

The following day, the counsellor contacted me to say that Billie hadn't shown up. I left a message, and in case she preferred to see a female doctor, left a time to come in and see one of my colleagues. But again, Billie didn't turn up.

I spoke with Simon and Amy: they were both furious with Billie, and thought her decision more about being wilful and obstinate than about expressing a genuine desire for motherhood. Otherwise, the pregnancy was going well: she had a touch of nausea, was sleeping more than usual, but was still making it in to school. Her parents thought that she was taking the folic acid I'd given. Billie was early in pregnancy for review by the midwives, but there was a new scheme – one-to-one support for teenage mums, throughout pregnancy and for the first couple of years. It was called the 'Family Nurse Partnership'; an idea planted in the United States in the early 1980s, recently sown in Scotland. Extra funding meant there was more midwife and nurse time to spend with the young pregnant women, and to support them. It encouraged healthier pregnancies, better language development for babies, better school outcomes for their mums, fewer subsequent pregnancies, and a dramatic improvement in keeping fathers engaged. The nurses and midwives of the scheme would liaise with Billie's teachers, and start preparing her for what it would be like to be heavily pregnant at thirteen, and care for a baby at fourteen.

The partnership arranged an ultrasound scan: the pregnancy was about twelve weeks on, and the baby a strong, healthy girl.

Billie was seen regularly by the nurses of the partnership, but eight weeks passed before I saw her back in clinic. Her lower back was beginning to hurt, she said, and she wanted a medical letter excusing her from gym class. 'How is it all going?' I asked.

'Fine,' she said, and for the first time in years looked directly at me.

'Did you have your twenty-week scan yet?'

'It was amazing,' she said, her face brightening. 'Sometimes I just can't believe that there's a new person inside, waiting to come out.' She put both hands on her belly, regarding it with an expression of fear mingled with pride. 'It's incredible when I can feel her moving inside me.'

'And your mum and dad? How are they getting used to the idea?'

Her face fell.

FOR MILLENNIA, knowledge about midwifery care must have been passed orally between women, but rarely written down. The few writings that have survived from the classical period, written by men, suggest they understood little about pregnancy. 'If a woman is pregnant with twins and either breast loses its fullness she will miscarry one,' says one of the Hippocratic treatises, 'if the right breast it will be the male child, or if the left, the female.' Some women *are* alerted they are going to miscarry by a sudden easing of breast tenderness, but in Hippocrates, that observation is conflated with senseless ideas about twins.

By the Middle Ages, manuals of midwifery began to show how babies might be positioned within the womb in late pregnancy, in order to give some guidance as to how they might be helped out. The images were schematic and poorly drawn, but they at least acknowledged that the growth of babies is not the stuff of miracles, but of material facts – a matter of anatomy and physiology. Men and women both were beginning to imagine what they might be feeling when they put their hands on a pregnant belly. One of the first to have useful images was an early sixteenth-century textbook called *The Byrth of Mankynde*, written by Eucharius Roesslin. It tabulated the different 'lies' of a baby in the womb, and offered advice about how best to deliver the baby in each case.

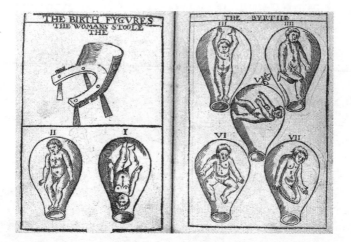

South of the Alps, Roesslin's contemporary Leonardo da Vinci was working on a far more accurate vision. Earlier in his career, he'd sketched out the ways in which he wanted to approach the mystery of new life and its development:

> ... begin with the conception of man, and [then] describe the nature of the womb and how the foetus lives in it, up to what stage it resides there, and in what way it quickens into life and feeds. Also its growth and what interval there is between one stage of growth and another. What it is that forces it out from the body of the mother.

Leonardo thought that a baby did not receive its own soul until birth ('the same soul governs the two bodies ... the things desired by the mother are often found impressed on the members of the child'), but others of his contemporaries believed it was somehow funnelled in from God at the 'quickening', when a pregnant woman began feeling movements within the womb – usually around twenty weeks. His *Study for the Foetus in the Womb* was made from a dissection he made of a woman who'd died at around this stage of pregnancy. Just as his images of coitus and conception prefigured those now obtainable with MRI scans, his images of the foetus in the womb are a hint of the 3D technology to come.

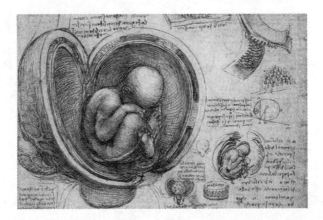

THE TRANSFORMATIONS OF PREGNANCY are as much social as physical: the pregnant woman's belly becomes a kind of unwilling public property, and her choices a matter of open debate. Strange hands assume licence to poke and prod; others may tut-tut disapprovingly if she dares drink coffee in public, never mind wine. Pregnancy illuminates with an unforgiving light how much society pries into women's bodies with more intensity, and with harsher judgement, than it does men's. Virginia Woolf skewered this disapproval in *Orlando*: 'the better to conceal the fact; the great fact; the only fact; but, nevertheless, the deplorable fact; which every modest woman did her best to deny until denial was impossible; the fact that she was about to bear a child'. But there's a flip side to the public scrutiny of pregnancy which manifests in a kind of wonder – a spellbound reification of the pregnant woman. For all our scientific understanding, an enchantment persists about new life forming within the body of another. Those intrusive hands may be hoping for some magic to rub off on them.

Margaret Atwood's *The Handmaid's Tale* describes a dystopian society in which fertility has plummeted, and women are subjugated as reproductive slaves. Atwood conveys both the sense of wonder that pregnancy inspires as well as the opprobrium meted out to many pregnant women. One of the captive women, Ofwarren, walks triumphantly into a shop frequented by the other handmaidens, her belly swollen like a 'huge fruit'. Ofwarren's hands lie over the dome of her abdomen as if protecting it, but also as if she hopes to absorb something of its vigour. The other women murmur excitedly; they long to touch her even as she glances haughtily at their own flat bellies. The tension in the room builds until one of the women mutters 'show-off'. Chitra Ramaswamy captures this strange mingling of admiration with resentment: 'How people stared, particularly women, with a deep, almost male gaze that bore an unnerving resemblance to lust,' she writes of the later stages of pregnancy. 'I began to realise that they weren't really looking at me at all. To be pregnant was to be a kind of mirror. Women, especially, wanted to see themselves in you.'

LEONARDO'S IMAGES of how the foetus lies in the womb weren't surpassed until the 1750s. The Scottish anatomist William Hunter saw the original folios among the Royal Collection in Windsor, and conceived an ambition to better them. Hunter was Queen Charlotte's personal physician, a celebrity doctor and a Fellow of the Royal Society. He recognised how much progress Leonardo had made towards comprehending the changes of pregnancy, but also how much more there still was to understand. With a Dutch illustrator called Jan van Rymsdyk, then famous in London circles for the grace and precision of his illustrations, he began work on his magnum opus, the anatomical work for which he's still best remembered: *The Anatomy of the Human Gravid Uterus*. Hunter had many enemies, was by report an insufferable narcissist, and was often accused of taking credit for others' work. Rymsdyk later said of him, 'it is a dishonest mean cunning, in making one self a great Man with other People's Merit'. But the work the two men created is one of clear-sighted vision, a fusion of Enlightenment science with an aesthetic sensibility reminiscent of the Dutch masters. It's a lesson in how scientific discovery can be a close cousin of art, and how much beauty can be revealed through anatomy.

The original drawings that Hunter made with Rymsdyk are held at the library of the University of Glasgow. I phoned ahead for an appointment – they're held in black, sepulchral boxes, and the staff need a few days' notice to bring them up from the archives. Each of the boxes needs its own table, and when they came up I saw that each was marked 'RESTRICTED'. Opening them, I found seventy-two drawings across thirty-four mounted plates. It was necessary to handle them with gloves, slowly lifting each image from the box as if unearthing them.

Hunter's interest was in relieving obstructed labour, and so his emphasis was on the final months of pregnancy. 'I was so fortunate as to meet with a Gravid Uterus,' he wrote cynically to a correspondent in February 1751, 'to which, from that time, all the hours have been dedicated.' The drawings are composed from about a score of these 'meetings'; they move backwards through a sequence of women prematurely dead, from full-term pregnancy to the days following conception. Rymsdyk's illustrations are of William Hunter's own dissections, as well as those of his brother John – the three men likely worked at times in the same space. Hunter's attitude to the dissected women is betrayed by his correspondence, and sounds shocking to modern ears. But in eighteenth-century London around one in fifty pregnancies ended in the mother's death. For Hunter, the death of a pregnant woman was routine; he was driven by scientific curiosity to understand pregnancy, but also by the imperative to reduce maternal deaths. Prints of engravings were produced for the education of clinicians all over the Anglophone world.

The Special Collections department of Glasgow University Library is on the twelfth floor; as I spread Rymsdyk's drawings across four tables I looked out over the city, and realised that I was within a few hundred yards of the lab where Ian Donald developed ultrasound. The foetal images hadn't faded; the babies were so lifelike it seemed scarcely possible they were drawn in death.

The printed edition of the engravings is dedicated to Hunter's sovereign George III, and attempts to impress upon the king the significance of his highly unconventional work:

> Sir, this work had no other claim to the honour with which it is distinguished by YOUR MAJESTY, than as

it illustrates one part of science hitherto imperfectly understood, it contains the foundation of another part of science, on which the lives and happiness of millions must depend.

Consistent with his interest in reducing maternal death, rather than understanding foetal development, Hunter often dismisses the baby with statements such as: 'The Foetus, with two turns of the navel-string round its neck, requires no explanation.' But Rymsdyk devotes great attention to the foetuses. Plate I shows the skin of the abdomen folded back like a mantle, the bulge of the womb filling the centre ground. Plate VI shows the same womb opened: a term baby in position, left arm extended, fingers curled as if plucking at strings. Her hair is stuck down with amniotic fluid as if sweating at the exertion of being born, or of dying.

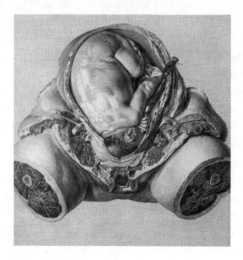

Plate XX shows a baby in breech position, fingertips touched lightly together. In one drawing made at around eighteen weeks of pregnancy, the detail is such that you can make out the window frame behind Rymsdyk, reflected on the shiny amniotic membrane. The membranes have been peeled back so carefully that the amniotic fluid is undisturbed; we look down with the artist on the baby floating in the liquid. Of this fluid, Hunter wrote: 'To the taste it is always very sensibly saltish: and a considerable quantity of common salt may be obtained by evaporating a large quantity of liquor' – like a fragment of the sea carried inside.

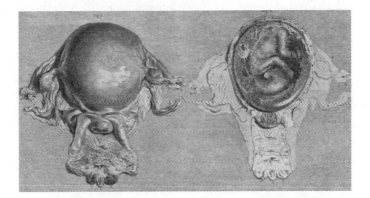

Some of the illustrations show the pelvis seen lengthways, like Leonardo's couple in coitus. Others have been drawn looking up at the swollen dome of the womb from between the thighs, as a midwife or obstetrician would gauge the progress of labour.

The final plate of Rymsdyk and Hunter's *The Anatomy of the Gravid Uterus* shows the sac of the embryo in reducing size – a shrinking crystal in a droplet of dew – retreating to its own conception.

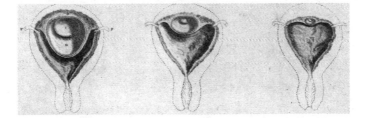

SIMON AND AMY came around to the idea of being grand-parents. Billie went into labour at forty-one weeks – only slightly overdue, but normal for a first pregnancy. She went through twenty-six hours of agony, a perineal tear, stitches, haemorrhage, transfusions, and delivery with the help of forceps. She might have appeared to have completed puberty, but her pelvis still had years to grow; if she'd lived a century earlier, she would almost certainly have died.

But she gave birth to a healthy baby girl, called the baby Danielle, and, as Amy had predicted, went back to school while Amy and Simon took on the job of being parents. I had déjà vu: Simon or Amy back regularly in clinic, a child bouncing on his or her knee, asking me about wheezes, fevers, rashes and feeding.

'It suits us you know, being a family of four,' Amy said to me one day, with Danielle in her arms. 'I didn't expect it to, but it does.'

'And Billie? How is she getting on?' I asked.

She shrugged. 'She plays with her a little bit, will pass me a nappy if I'm in the middle of changing her, but she never speaks about the pregnancy. It's like it never happened.' She looked down at Danielle, smiled at her and tickled her toes. 'I'm keeping a close eye on this one though,' she said; 'I don't want to be back here in a few years with a great-grandchild.'

14

Gigantism: Two Giants of Turin

Really, there must be some energizing element in the air here – to be
at home here will make one king of Italy.

Friedrich Nietzsche, Selected Letters

TURIN: A NORTHERN ITALIAN, French-inflected city of boulevards, *settecento* palaces, varnished wood and polished
brass; of plane trees, promenades and the river Po. Of Alps
visible on three horizons, Primo Levi's suicide, and Friedrich Nietzsche's madness. Before his breakdown Nietzsche
wrote of it: 'Here day after day dawns with the same bound-
less perfection and plenitude of sun: the glorious foliage in
glowing yellow, the sky and the big river delicately blue, the
air of greatest purity ... In every way, life is worth living
here.'

Turin's Museum of Human Anatomy is behind an
inconspicuous wooden door off one of the city's grandest
boulevards, up three flights of marble stairs. There are no
windows; the smells are of floor polish and plaster, with
a hint of formalin. Columns of stone are interleaved with
vitrines of dark lacquered wood. I worked once in Edinburgh's Anatomical Museum, arranging collections of
specimens for display, and Turin's museum felt familiar.
It too was built up in the 1800s, by obsessive categorisers

– part educational institute, part wonder-house. Skulls of Etruscans jostle with the skulls of apes. There are pickled hands and feet; twenty feet of coiled, preserved intestine; decapitated Peruvian mummies; wax models of the female pelvis with an erotic attention to detail. As in Edinburgh, phrenology heads sit side by side with the death masks of celebrities; wax models illustrate the development of the embryonic heart. Both museums are preoccupied with comparative anatomy – the natural world ransacked in the attempt to conjure order from the commotion of Life.

In Edinburgh, you're met at the door by the skeleton of a hanged murderer,* and in Turin you're met by the skeleton of a giant. Giacomo Borghello of Liguria was seven feet two inches tall when he died in 1829, at just nineteen years old. The plaque didn't mention it, but I asked the attendant how he died: he'd been employed in a circus, she said, and his cause of death was given as 'heart failure'. Borghello's mortal remains, yellowed as parchment, are suspended in a cabinet, and my head reached not much higher than his pelvis. His skull was undersized in comparison with his gigantic limbs, and the growth plates ('epiphyses') at the end of each long bone were not even beginning to fuse. Something was driving Borghello's enormous growth even as it killed him.

The attendants of Turin's museum wouldn't allow it, but I would have liked to glance inside his skull, just between and behind the eyes, at the place where the pituitary gland nestles. The pituitary produces the hormone that drives growth; the recess in the skull where it fits is named the *sella turcica* or 'Turkish saddle', because early modern anatomists noticed its similarity to the high-pommelled saddles of the Ottoman cavalry. In producing so much growth hormone Borghello's pituitary was likely to

---

* William Hare, of 'Burke and Hare', who were paid for their murder victims by the Edinburgh anatomist Robert Knox.

have been swollen, and his *sella turcica* wider than usual to accommodate it.*

IN TURIN I ALSO WENT to visit Piazza Carlo Alberto, where the philosopher Nietzsche lived in the late 1880s: 'the only suitable place for me,' he said of it; 'it shall be my home henceforward'. On one of the piazza's corners I found a laudatory plaque, erected on the centenary of Nietzsche's birth. Engraved in marble, it was a hymn to gigantism of the mind: 'In this house Friedrich Nietzsche knew the fullness of spirit that tempts the unknown, the will to dominion that calls forth the hero.'

Nietzsche wrote his autobiography *Ecce Homo* in Turin, during three frantic weeks in October and November of 1888.† In it, he describes feeling as heroic as a polar explorer: 'The ice is near, the solitude is terrible – but how peacefully all things lie in the light! How freely one breathes!' Nietzsche saw himself as a giant among dwarves: *Ecce Homo* has section headings called 'Why I am so wise', 'Why I am so clever', 'Why I write such excellent books'.

Nietzsche felt that it was his duty as a philosopher to encourage mankind to expand perspective and strive to become *Übermensch*, variously translated as 'Overman', 'Beyond-man' or 'Superman'. These 'supermen' included philosophers such as Montaigne and Aristotle, and were rare in the history of humanity. Nietzsche imagined them as fellow members of a 'republic of creative minds', 'each giant calling to his brother through the desolate intervals of time ... undisturbed by the wanton noises of the dwarfs that creep past beneath them'.

In a section of what he considered his finest work, *Thus*

---

* Pituitary' means 'snot'; early anatomists thought that the gland channelled mucus.

† 'Ecce Homo' are Pontius Pilate's words on releasing Jesus of Nazareth to the mob: 'Behold The Man'.

Spake Zarathustra, a thinly disguised Nietzsche carries a dwarf up a mountain to show him the breadth and nobility of his vision. The dwarf finds the vision incomprehensible. Nietzsche makes an explicit correlation between exalted physical stature and exalted mental perspective, then compares that exaltation with the tininess of most human concerns. He seems to be refuting the old saying, repeated by scholars from the twelfth-century John of Salisbury to Isaac Newton, that academics are simply dwarves who see far 'because they have stood on the shoulders of giants'. On the contrary, Nietzsche maintained that he could see far because he was a giant of the mind.

In the autumn of 1888 Nietzsche wrote of 'a supreme feeling of pride which nothing could equal', articulating his sense of 'the disparity which obtains between the greatness of my task, and the smallness of my contemporaries.' His expansive sense of himself and his mission continued to grow.

THE PITUITARY GLAND is the strategic command of several of the body's hormonal systems: it is essential not only for growth but also for healing, sex, birth, lactation, response to trauma and maintenance of equilibrium. It sits on the margins between body and brain. In the embryo, the gland begins as a pouch at the back of the throat; it migrates up and back into its saddle-like position beneath the cranial vault between week four and week six of gestation. There it takes in nerves, and fuses with a small outgrowth from the brain that becomes its posterior half.

Through secretion of TSH, or 'thyroid stimulating hormone', the pituitary controls the body's metabolic rate by calibrating the release of thyroxine, another hormone, from a gland in the neck. Failure of the gland to respond is the cause of one of the more common hormonal transformations: with an underactive thyroid we gain weight, lose hair, feel sluggish and shiver with cold in a warm room.

With an overactive thyroid the converse is true: we lose weight, tremble with agitation and feel hot even in a cold room. The thyroid is intimately connected to how active we are – in ancient Rome, mothers would allegedly measure the neck circumference of their daughters after they'd spent an evening with a man, because sexual encounters cause the gland to swell.

The pituitary also secretes LH and FSH, 'luteinizing hormone' and 'follicle stimulating hormone', which control the testes and ovaries, sexual differentiation, ovulation and the generation of sperm. Through prolactin the pituitary drives the production of milk in the breasts (among other things) and through ACTH, 'adrenocorticotrophic hormone', it controls the production of natural steroids. But it is the pituitary's secretion of growth hormone that drives the lengthening of bones and determines the height we attain.

The response of the long bones to growth hormone is time-limited – once the growth plates have fused at the close of puberty, they ignore the pituitary's command to grow. But if the pituitary gland goes on producing growth hormone after fusion of the growth plates, other parts of the body can still respond: the heart thickens and blood pressure rises, the jaw lengthens, the forehead becomes embossed, the hands, feet and nose swell. This constellation of changes is called 'acromegaly', or 'swelling of the extremities'. It may come as a consequence of untreated gigantism in adolescence, or it may arise in adulthood, if production of growth hormone surges (usually due to a pituitary tumour) later in life.

The transformation of acromegaly happens so slowly that for the most part it's hardly noticed by close family and friends – usually it's only after an absence of months that the change becomes obvious. But those familiar with its distinctive features may spot it at once: I knew a hormone specialist who recognised evolving acromegaly in the barista from whom he bought his morning coffee. The barista handed over his coffee one morning, and my colleague handed over a business card and, scrawled on it, a clinic appointment.

Since the mid-twentieth century it's been technically possible to treat both acromegaly and gigantism with either surgery to the pituitary gland or drugs to block growth hormone's effects – or both. It's necessary too: Borghello's heart wasn't unusual in giving out at nineteen, overwhelmed by the challenge of pumping blood to such a colossal frame, while being pathologically thickened both by growth hormone itself and by his elevated blood pressure. A swollen pituitary can cause other problems, such as blindness, which is caused by the squeezing of the optic nerves. It's as if, as human beings, our stature is calibrated to stay within a particular range. Beyond that range, life becomes difficult to sustain.

IN *ECCE HOMO*, Nietzsche wrote that he felt 'certain at each moment of my immortality'. It was to be among his last writings. On 3 January 1889 he came upon a horse being flogged just a few yards from his front door on Piazza Carlo Alberto. He rushed to embrace and protect it, then fell sobbing, arms around the horse's neck, before being carried back to his quarters by his landlord. Over subsequent days he wrote a series of crazed letters to his usual correspondents, including Richard Wagner's wife Cosima ('Ariadne, I love you'), and Fräulein von Salis ('The world is transfigured, for God is on earth. Do you not see how all the heavens rejoice? I have just now taken possession of my kingdom, am casting the Pope into prison'). He signed these letters as 'Dionysus' or 'the crucified one'. Franz Overbeck, a Protestant theologian and close friend, recognised that Nietzsche's customary arrogance had given way to something more sinister, so he came to Turin and arranged to transfer him to an asylum in Basel.

In Basel, Nietzsche shuffled between psychiatric clinics

and his mother's house for a decade, before succumbing to pneumonia, probably precipitated by a series of strokes. His madness has variously been attributed to syphilis, bipolar illness, a benign brain tumour, and a disorder of the cerebral arteries. He never again wrote anything of significance. It was as if the will to dominate, to be a giant among dwarves, contained within it the catalyst for his own destruction.

OPPOSITE BORGHELLO'S SKELETON in Turin there is a diminutive skeleton with all its growth plates fused: not the skeleton of a child, but an adult with arrested growth. The museum's description reads '*un esempio di nanismo armonico*' – 'an example of harmonic dwarfism'; though small, the body is in standard if childlike proportion. In life, this individual lacked the human growth hormone of which Borghello had a surfeit.

Within flexible limits society gives advantage to those who are bullish and self-confident, as it does to those who are above average height. In his book *Size Matters*, the science journalist Stephen Hall comments on his own experience as a man of five feet five and three-quarter inches: we live in an altocracy. Hall quotes the perspective of an eighteenth-century German physician, Johann Augustin Stoller: 'Nobility of soul accompanies tallness of body.' Sociologists tell us that tall people are consistently deemed more intelligent, congenial, reliable and authoritative, and Hall points out that in US presidential elections, the taller of the two candidates usually wins.*

Once a patient of mine who lived on one of the wealthiest streets in Edinburgh brought her daughter to my clinic to request referral to a growth specialist. 'She's stopped growing, and she's only five foot,' she said. Molly had been the first in her class to enter puberty, and now, aged

---

* There are exceptions: George W. Bush managed to beat John Kerry, and Jimmy Carter beat Gerald Ford.

fourteen, was being overtaken by all of her classmates. Both her parents were below average height.

When people believe modern medicine to be capable of miracles, I try to take it as testimony of just how accustomed we have become to its success. But I had to tell her that, in this case, medicine had nothing to offer: 'There's nothing wrong,' I told Molly as kindly as I could, 'and no reason for a referral.' I plotted out her height on a centile chart and showed her where she stood: 'The height at which you stop growing is related to your own parents' heights, your nutrition in childhood, and your age at puberty. If you start the growth spurt of puberty early, you stop growing earlier too.' Even if growth hormone had been indicated it was now too late – the growth plates of Molly's long bones were already beginning to fuse.*

The use of growth hormones as a treatment for short stature has had the unintended effect of medicalising natural variation in height. Growth hormone secretion from the pituitary gland peaks at night, and treatment with artificial hormone is given as an injection under the skin every evening, within an hour of going to bed. In those who most need it the effect can be dramatic: one or two inches may be gained within six months of treatment, and one or two shoe sizes.

Until the 1980s, the hormone was extracted from the pituitary glands of cadavers, but it's now synthesised artificially in the laboratory. Even so, the process is complex and sophisticated – human growth hormone is one of the most expensive treatments in medicine. At the time of writing, a course may cost three or four times the average UK annual salary, and those with a normally functioning pituitary can expect to gain an inch in height at best. But if Hall is right, and height is so directly correlated to economic success, then

---

* Though as discussed in 'Puberty', her pelvis would still have some years to grow.

even the vast costs of human growth hormone treatment could prove a worthwhile (if ethically dubious) investment.

TO BE PERSUADED to leave Turin, Nietzsche had to be drugged with sedatives, and cajoled into believing that Switzerland was putting on a state visit in celebration of his new royal status. On the train north he sang songs and proclaimed himself king of Italy.*

If only he'd paid more attention to some of his favourite philosophers: Aristotle believed that virtue lay in finding the balance between extremes; Montaigne warned against hankering after physical or intellectual stature. One of Montaigne's famous essays, 'Of Moderation', advises human beings to stay within 'the fair and beaten way that nature has traced for us'. He suggests temperance even in philosophy, and offers a passage that could stand as a critique of Nietzsche's own grandiloquent claims: 'In the end [philosophy] renders a man brutish and vicious, a condemner of religion and the common laws.' In another essay he warns against an obsessive preoccupation with height: 'A man of low stature is as much a man as a giant; neither men nor their lives are measured by the ell.'

---

* Overbeck says that he sang the 'wonderfully beautiful gondola song' reproduced in *Ecce Homo*: 'And my soul, a stringed instrument,/ Sang, touched by invisible hands,/ To itself a secret gondola song,/ Trembling with all the colours of bliss.' See also *Selected Letters of Friedrich Nietzsche*, Christopher Middleton, trans., p. 354.

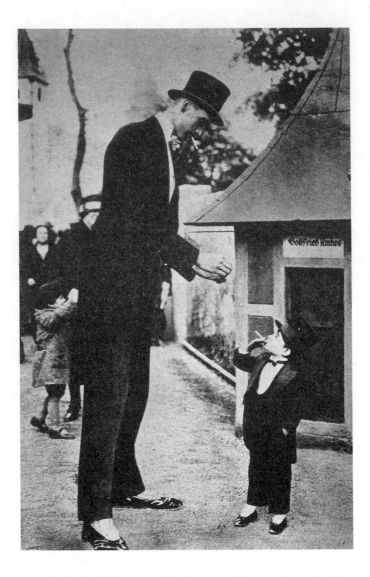

15

Gender: The Two Lives of Tiresias

We must acknowledge this Androgynal condition in man.

Thomas Browne, *Pseudodoxia Epidemica*

AT MEDICAL SCHOOL in the mid-1990s, my paediatric training took place in a Victorian hospital in Edinburgh called
the 'Sick Kids'. But it began before birth, so to speak, in the
modern maternity unit a short stroll away across the park.
It was there in the obstetric hospital that I was obliged to
learn how to deliver babies, as well as gain an understanding of the many perils that attend the first few minutes of
life. When I'd been signed off as competent to assist births,
the next stage in training followed the newborn babies into
an adjoining neonatal unit.

The babies we admitted were often mortally ill and
critically underweight, but one day there was an unusual
admission: a perfectly healthy nine-pound newborn. In
the moments after birth, when its parents had cried out to
ask if it was a boy or a girl, the midwife had gasped, 'I
don't know!' The baby had ambiguous genitalia, a small
penis as well as a vagina. He or she was robust and feeding
well – no metabolic or hormonal problems were causing
the ambiguity. The only reason to stay in the hospital was
to figure out whether 'she' really was a 'he', or vice versa.

The importance placed on the distinction was implicit even in the name bands we wrapped around the babies' wrists. These were usually colour-coded pink or blue, but the new baby was given one of white. The parents were anxious and bewildered, and only became more so when the attending neonatologist began to speak of blood tests, scans and gonadal biopsies.

Later that day, I walked back across the park to the library at the Sick Kids and looked up 'Disorders of sexual differentiation' in the textbooks. 'Ambiguity of the external genitalia at the time of birth causes great distress for the parents,' I read. 'Sensitive explanation is vital.' It was estimated that one in 2,000 babies manifest some degree of genital ambiguity, and as regards the tests: 'Complete diagnostic evaluation requires special expertise as it has to consider the long-term functional role of the individual as well as the precise gender.' The book went on to explain that the vast majority of babies with ambiguous genitalia fall into two broad groups. Intersex babies could turn out to be genetically female – with two X chromosomes – but their clitorises had swelled to the size of small penises because of a hormonal condition generating unusually high levels of testosterone-like hormones (androgens) while still in the womb. But there were also genetic males – possessing an X and a Y chromosome – whose developing genitalia had proven partially insensitive to testosterone, or who hadn't been able to generate adequate amounts of the hormone to physically differentiate. As human beings, our default form is female – if the bodies of XY babies don't sense androgens in their blood, they develop short, blind-ended vaginas with a clitoris instead of a penis.

There was a third category in the textbook – 'true hermaphrodites': these were babies born with both testicular and ovarian tissue, and small penises as well as wombs and vaginas. Highly improbable events had to coincide for this to happen, and there were several ways in which it could come about. The most likely is that a 'male' sperm carrying a single 'Y' chromosome, and a 'female' sperm carrying a single 'X' chromosome, fertilise an egg that has just divided, then those two fertilised eggs fuse together. The bodily tissues of these 'true hermaphrodites' are a tessellation of male and female cells, and are known in medical jargon as 'mosaics'. Mosaicism has been known since at least the 1930s, but it wasn't until the late 1950s that it was realised this phenomenon could lead to hermaphroditism.

The textbook said, in clear but insensitive style, that 'a genetic male with functioning testes but feminized external genitalia is better reared as a girl.' I wondered how they could be so sure.

It took a few days to sort out all the blood tests and scans – days in which the parents, in the interests of neutrality, referred to the baby as Sam. Names might tolerate ambiguity, but the deeply gendered nature of language meant that no one could figure out which pronouns to use. 'It' seemed grossly insensitive, but 'he' or 'she' might prove incorrect.* Sam was gloriously oblivious, breastfeeding well and putting on weight.

When all the results were put together, they implied that Sam had rare, 'true' hermaphroditism: a mosaic of male and female cells had given rise to elements of both sexes. As well as a penis and vagina, Sam had a womb as well as a fallopian tube leading from an ovary on the left side, but on the right there was a buried testicle, and a vas deferens, the duct that in adulthood conveys sperm from the testicle to the urethra.

In the 1990s in Edinburgh, there wasn't a great deal of sensitivity around gender ambiguity, and the possibility of raising Sam as neither male nor female – being dressed in green or red instead of pink or blue – didn't appear to arise.

---

* The Italian poet Carlo Emilio Gadda pronounced pronouns 'the lice of thought' for the lazy thinking they introduce.

The very nature of the English language seemed to demand a decision. 'She's a girl,' Sam's mother decided finally, once we had explained the findings of the tests, 'Sam is Samantha.' What would be done about her penis was left for a later decision. Her bald little head was immediately decorated with a flowery headband. Her cot-side filled up with pink cards, frilly blankets, and heart-shaped balloons.

SAM WAS LIVING, thriving proof that there's more to men and women than X and Y chromosomes, but modern western culture, and in particular western medicine, often struggles with ambiguity and androgyny. Through most of the twentieth century, medical orthodoxy held to the line articulated in my paediatric textbook: boys without male genitals (absent either because of a developmental anomaly, or consequent to an accident) could simply be raised as girls. But it was increasingly noted that in adolescence, many of these individuals began to express discomfort with the gender allocated to them. Early hormonal exposure seemed to have a role in determining later identity. It was noticed, too, that XX babies raised as boys because of their enlarged clitorises reported high levels of preference for identifying as women. One study from 2005 put this proportion at 12 per cent, while the proportion of XY babies raised as girls, but who later identified as male, was lower at 5 per cent.

Modern medicine is only now getting to grips with these fluid ideas of gender identity, but thousands of years ago, in the philosophy and mythology of the Greeks, these concepts were already being explored. Plato's *Symposium* tells of the contribution of the playwright Aristophanes to an earnest discussion about love. In the beginning there were three sexes, he says, not two: male, female and androgynous. Each consisted of four hands, four feet, two sets of genitals and two faces gazing in opposite directions. Those beings wholly male came from the sun, those all female came from the earth, and those in whom male and female parts coexisted came from the moon.

All three groups of these original, powerful beings began to threaten the gods, so Zeus split them down the middle 'as you might divide an egg with a hair', doubling their numbers but condemning each to search forever for his or her other half. Those who were once androgynous became heterosexuals, useful for breeding but prone to adultery. Those who were all-woman became lesbians and those who were all-man became homosexual men ('the best of boys and youths, for they have the most manly nature'). Aristophanes was a comic playwright, and seems to have anticipated being mocked for his ideas. 'This is my discourse of love,' he says in the *Symposium*, 'which, although different to yours, I must beg you to leave unassailed by the shafts of your ridicule.'

From the ancient world through to the Renaissance, there are plenty of examples in medical and other writings in which men and women are thought of less as opposites than as sharing essential characteristics, and capable of changing sides. From the anatomies of Aristotle and Galen, to the speculations of Thomas Browne, for most of scientific history, transition between female and male was thought of not just as possible but as expected from time to time. Only about 200 or 300 years ago, with the hardening rationalism of the Enlightenment, did this fluidity give way.

Another Greek story, the myth of the prophet Tiresias, attests to a fascination with gender flexibility. As a young man, Tiresias was walking in the forest when he came upon a pair of mating snakes – a symbol of bisexuality and an omen of ill luck. Instead of rushing away from the misfortune, 'he struck them across their backs'. The female snake was killed, and Tiresias was transformed instantly into a woman. Snakes were symbolic of transformation because they periodically shed their skins, and in her new skin Tiresias became a prostitute in Thebes, and later a mother.

After seven years, she came upon mating snakes again, and this time struck the male, and was promptly returned to male form.

Ovid follows the tale of Tiresias with a bawdy, barroom story about Zeus and his wife Hera having an argument over whether men or women had the greatest pleasure during sex. As the only ancient transsexual, Tiresias was called in to adjudicate, and testified that if sexual pleasure consists of ten parts then women enjoy nine-tenths and man enjoys one part only. It's an odd tale, and given the assertion that only about one-third of women in western culture reach climax during heterosexual intercourse, perhaps says more about male anxieties than it does about sexual realities.

TARIK TOLD ME that he had known from a young age that he should have been born a girl. He was neither straight nor gay, and he couldn't remember ever being interested in sex. As a boy, he'd been more interested in Barbie than in Action Man, and was scolded for wearing his sister's dresses. Outwardly he had been a calm and studious child, but a whirlwind of anxieties over his gender identity gathered force through adolescence. He became an academic, and when we met three or four years ago, he was just beginning a long research sabbatical. The free time offered by the sabbatical had given him his first opportunity to think about changing his gender identity. 'You're the first person I've told,' he told me, sobbing. 'I can't go on like this.'

Since my time in medical school, neurodevelopmental research had moved on: momentum had gathered against the proposition that a boy without a penis should simply be raised as a girl – and vice versa. Elements of gender differentiation are deeply rooted in the brain and in hormones – there's little doubt now that there's more to a sense of gender identity than socialisation. Twin studies imply that the incidence of discontent with birth gender is higher in identical twins than it is in fraternal (non-identical) twins, which implies at least a partial genetic component. Other studies have found that chromosomal disorders that lead to reduced testosterone production in boys may result in increased desire for male-to-female transition.

Until recently, gender variance was considered a deviance. The first Diagnostic and Statistical Manual ('DSM') of the American Psychiatric Association, published in 1952, placed gender variance under the blunt heading 'Sexual Deviation'. The second manual, published in 1968, retained the same classification, although by then the Kinsey Report on sexual behaviour in the United States had broadened awareness of sexual diversity. The third DSM, from 1980, created the new category 'Gender Identity Disorders', which was carried over into the fourth, from 1994. The fifth version, in 2013, has switched the term 'disorder' for 'dysphoria' – a state of mind that connotes suffering and distress. This term, too, has been criticised as excluding those entirely at ease in their adopted gender, and the more neutral term 'variance' is now proposed.

Tarik was profoundly dysphoric; every morning he woke with a plunging feeling in his gut, knowing he faced another day of acting as a man. He was depressed, and his sleep was agitated and unrefreshing. His body disgusted him, particularly his chest hair and beard, his jaw line, penis and scrotum. He could barely bring himself to touch his genitals and found it easier to wash them quickly, in the dark.

Medical guidelines in both the UK and the US require living fully in the 'adopted gender role' for twelve months or more before gender reassignment surgery. 'I hate that expression, "living in a role",' Tarik told me when we began to discuss transition. 'For me, this is living authentically.' With support from a local gender identity clinic he took the difficult step of telling his academic colleagues, his parents and his siblings, and began to live as 'Teresa'.

Tiresias had switched gender at the strike of a snake

– with the support of the clinic, I began the much slower process of effecting a comparable metamorphosis with prescription drugs. The first drug was finasteride, which inhibits the generation of the most potent form of testosterone within the body. It's used to shrink the prostate, and in small doses it helps to retard male-pattern baldness. This was only partially successful – it isn't a very effective treatment – and gave way after a few months to leuprorelin injections, initially monthly and then, once her body was used to them, once every three months. Leuprorelin inhibits the pituitary gland's production of gonad-stimulating hormones and can shrivel the testes – it has the potential to cause flushing of the skin, a collapse of interest in sex and weakening of the bones. A few weeks after leuprorelin was established, we commenced oestrogen therapy. This feminises the body and promotes the development of breasts, but can bring on blood clots as well as subtly increase the risks of stroke, heart attack and breast cancer.

This all took a couple of years, and the final phase of transition to Teresa would be the most difficult: surgical removal of the testicles and parts of the penis, and then the creation of a blind-ended vagina using the penile skin. The physical transition proceeded in two stages – Teresa's convalescence from each procedure took months. The body's own power of healing can rebel against its new form: initially, trans women have to keep their newly created vagina open with the daily use of dilators, and regular douching with antiseptic solution. Parts of the scrotal skin are infolded and sutured down to resemble labia.

Once Teresa's physical scars had healed, her dysphoria was replaced by euphoria. She went back to her position at the university and the quiet, studious life she'd had before transition. She told me that her academic work was better than it had ever been. Oestrogen affects more than just the shape and hair distribution of the body: 'My brain loves these hormones,' another trans woman told me shortly after commencing oestrogen therapy. 'It feels as if a missing cog has fallen into place.' Teresa remained uninterested in sex or in finding a partner. There were still immense challenges she faced: teasing and disapproval from her colleagues; disappointment and disbelief from her parents; harassment in the street; the need for ongoing hormonal treatment; her ceaseless battle with chest and facial hair. But her sleep now was restful, and the feeling of dread on awakening had gone.

EVEN THIRTY YEARS AGO the transition from Tarik to Teresa would have been improbable: gender surgery was far more difficult to access, and it was rudimentary in terms of the procedures that could be offered. But though the science and the surgery to effect gender transition is a relatively recent phenomenon, classical medical ideas of gender and sexual differentiation prefigured it. They hinged on the assumption that male bodies were simply warmer than those of women, and the temperature of your mother's womb determined whether you'd develop male or female sexual organs. According to Galen, these organs were fundamentally the same: the scrotum was simply a womb turned inside out, and the penis was an extruded vagina. To transform a woman to a man, all that was necessary was to heat the pelvic organs, which would then 'break free' and become externalised. It was an absurd view in many respects, but it did allow for the possibility that gender exists on a spectrum, and that we all carry the potential for transformation.

This idea persisted from classical times to the medieval, and endured past the Renaissance. The sixteenth-century French philosopher Michel de Montaigne and his surgeon contemporary Ambroise Paré both tell the story of a female swineherd, Marie, who, while energetically jumping a ditch after some pigs, found that her vagina had 'extruded' into a penis, making her a man. The transformation was confirmed by a bishop and Marie was re-baptised 'Germain', and honoured by being made one of the king's courtiers. It seems as if Germain was welcomed in his new form because he'd transitioned through an apparent act of God, rather than through his own choice. It's likely that Germain was an XY male, and the growth of his penis was not sudden but took place gradually over months; he probably had a hormonal condition that had diminished the conversion of testosterone to its most potent form, and so developed feminine genitalia in the womb. The sequence is well described by the heroine/hero of Jeffrey Eugenides's novel *Middlesex*: the heightened hormonal boost of puberty causes the growth of a penis and beard, descent of the testicles, as well as a deepening of the voice. This particular genetic condition is also relatively common in a genetically restricted community in the Dominican Republic, where those who experience it are known as *hue-vedoces*, or 'testicles at twelve'.

Montaigne tells another gender transition story, about a woman called Mary who took to living as a man. Mary became a weaver in a distant town and fell in love with a woman whom he married, and with whom he lived 'for four or five months, to [his wife's] satisfaction'. But then someone from his home town recognised him and called in the authorities, who tried him as a woman. Mary was hanged for 'using illicit devices to supply her defect in sex'. In the French society of the period, acts of God were permissible, but Mary's transition was perceived as a matter of wanton choice.

In 1931 a German physician named Felix Abraham published a description of a new procedure, carried out by a Dr Gohrbandt in Berlin, on two individuals with gender dysphoria. The first, Dora R., had tried repeatedly as a boy to amputate his penis. Abraham described the second, Toni E., as a 'homosexual' and 'transvestite' who had only ever felt comfortable in women's clothing. Toni E. was fifty-two at the time of her surgery – Abraham adds that she had waited until the death of her wife before proceeding.*

Gohrbandt's 'vaginoplasty' procedure involved the creation of a tunnel through the pelvic muscles from the perineum up to the abdominal lining. The new cavity was then packed with a rubber sponge coated with skin grafts taken from the thigh. Abraham concluded his case reports with a summary of his case for facilitating surgical transition:

> One could raise an objection to this type of surgery, that it is some kind of luxury surgery with a frivolous character, because the patient possibly will return to the doctor after some time with new and greater demands. This cannot be excluded. It was not easy for us to decide on the described procedures, but the patients were not to be dismissed, but also were in a mental state that made it probable that self-mutilation, with life-endangering complications, could be possible. From other cases we have learned that transvestites [sic] indeed cause themselves very severe harm if the doctor does not fulfil their wishes.

Following the simple vaginoplasty of Gohrbandt, it wasn't until the 1950s that Dr Georges Burou in Morocco began to use inversion of the penile skin to create a vagina – a neater, and from the perspective of healing, more successful method of vaginoplasty. Hundreds of trans women are said to have passed through Burou's clinic through the 1960s and 1970s. 'I do not transform men into women,' he announced in 1973. 'I transform male genitals into genitals that have a feminine aspect. All the rest is in the patient's head.'

---

* The same year Lili Elbe, a trans woman born in Denmark who changed her name from Einar Wegener, died from surgical complications of a procedure to implant a womb in her pelvis.

In a sense, Burou could be said to have been correct: it's now known that there are structures in the brain, constituting parts of the hormonal and emotional regulatory systems, that exhibit differences between the sexes. A postmortem study from Holland found that the hypothalamus of trans women shared neuronal characteristics with natal women. Whether these similarities pre-date or post-date the surgical transition (i.e. whether they were innate or consequent to behavioural or hormonal changes) wasn't clarified by the study. But either way, in their 'heads' and in their 'brains', the trans women were identifiably women.

There is much still unknown about gender, sexuality and the developing brain. It's becoming apparent that there are critical moments in the womb that determine whether we grow up identifying as male, female or somewhere in between, and neuronal structures within the brain come to reflect these different positions. This isn't to deny that the expression of identity is enormously influenced by our individual contexts and cultures, or to contest the evident truth that elements of our identities shift ceaselessly through different social interactions.

The next few years are going to see a gathering appreciation of the many determining factors involved in the expression of gender identity, as well as improvements in surgical techniques. Many elements of transition thought impossible are now looking achievable: uterine transplants have become technically possible, and in 2014 a recipient of such a transplant gave birth. Though no trans woman has yet successfully received a uterine transplant, many have expressed the wish to do so, and it would be surprising if one isn't announced within the next few years.

As a doctor, my role is to ease suffering and promote health; my interest in gender reassignment (or 'confirmation' as many trans men and women prefer it) is primarily whether it eases the distress of the patient consulting me, and helps them live their lives. Gender variance holds a mirror up to the polarisation of gender in our society, which instructs us relentlessly and emphatically to *choose*. It's known now that forcing this choice can be harmful, and isn't backed up by the scientific evidence – we all benefit from allowing elements of our identity to be in flux. In her book *The Argonauts*, Maggie Nelson quotes her partner's impatience with the idea that anyone with an ambiguous expression of gender must be on a journey to one binary extreme or the other ('I'm not on my way anywhere'), and points out that all of us are in ceaseless transition, irrespective of gender: 'on the inside, we were two human animals undergoing transformation beside each other, bearing each other loose witness. In other words, we were aging.'

There is a gathering movement of people who feel that, for them, gender reassignment surgery may have been a mistake – that the medical profession's checks and barriers to hormonal and surgical transition, though formidable, were for them insufficient. After twenty years living as a woman, 'Elan Anthony' detransitioned, like Tiresias, back to being a man. He calls his journey 'third way trans'. 'I couldn't bond with people and eventually started therapy to work on why I couldn't have relationships and why my body was so tense,' he said in an interview with *The Guardian*. 'I eventually realised that a lot of this had to do with trying to present myself as female, which was unnatural for my body.' He'd been bullied as a boy, feeling himself at the bottom of a strict male hierarchy; through therapy he came to realise that his childhood identification as female reflected an unconscious need to escape. One of the greatest barriers faced by Elan was criticism within the trans community: 'It is difficult being part of the psychological community that is so pro-transition right now, and being one of the few critics,' he said, 'but it feels like there are a lot more people speaking out about detransition, as well as more clinicians who are interested in looking at alternative ways to deal with dysphoria.'

When in *The Waste Land* T. S. Eliot wrote of the pain of being trapped between two lives, tortured and unable to be fully accepted in either, the allegorical figure he chose was Tiresias, 'throbbing between two lives'. To undergo transition from one gender to another takes courage and determination, but in a polarised culture, so too does the occupation of an ambiguous, androgynous space. In the natural world, to occupy a space part-way between two genders is not just possible, it's common. The testimony from science, medicine and people with fluid or ambiguous gender all indicate that the distance between Tiresias's two lives needn't be so great, and that sometimes the choice need not be quite so stark.

16

Jetlag: The Brain that Holds the Sky

The brain is wider than the sky,
For, put them side by side,
The one the other will include
With ease, and you beside.

Emily Dickinson

ON THE ANTARCTIC RESEARCH STATION where I lived as base doctor for a year there were almost four months of sunlessness, while the planet's winter tilt put the continent in shadow. But it wasn't perpetually dark: there was plenty to see and the sky was always changing.* On emerging from Halley base I became accustomed to looking up and seeing the wheel of the stars and planets, meteor showers, or the slow creep of satellites. The ice was usually moonlit, and at that latitude there were weekly and sometimes daily auroras, granting depth and spectacular brilliance to the sky. On midwinter's day, almost two months into the dark time, we added another source of light – we lit a fire. We piled up wooden packing crates and set them ablaze.

---

* I wrote about my year on the station in *Empire Antarctica: Ice, Silence & Emperor Penguins* (London: Chatto, 2012).

To warm yourself by a bonfire built on ice is a distinctive experience. The floating ice shelf beneath our feet was hundreds of metres thick, fixed to the shoreline, and composed of snow that had fallen further into Antarctica over millennia, and then flowed slowly, as a glacier, out over the Weddell Sea. As the fire gathered intensity, the compacted snow melted and seeped away, the flames sinking their own firepit deeper into the oblivious ice. To the south of the base we could see the contours of the continent rising towards the South Pole, its immense weight settling beneath the stars and auroras as if in obeisance. On midwinter's night we kept our backs to it, holding our beer bottles towards the fire to keep them from freezing. For a few hours we bathed in heat and light, trying not to think how alien an environment we were living in, and how far we were from those we loved.

For some, the winter so far had been particularly tough. Sleep had become restless and unrefreshing: as *Homo sapiens* we're best adapted to the rhythms of tropical skies, and the lack of sunlight month after month was sending our body clocks awry. Some of my base-mates experienced 'free-running', when the body's internal rhythm loses its purchase on the celestial twenty-four-hour clock and slips to a shorter, or longer, internal timer. Free-running can lead to a bewildering, exhausting sensation of perpetual jetlag, as the body tries to run to a rhythm shorter, or longer, than twenty-four hours.

The body's internal clock is called 'circadian' (Latin for 'almost a day') and is characterised by the secretion of melatonin at night from the pineal gland of the brain. When we're in temperate or tropical latitudes, the pineal's own rhythms are calibrated by the sky's alternation of light with dark. Deprived of natural light during a polar winter, the pineal gland of those who by nature are early-rising larks defaults to a shorter internal 'day' of just twenty-two or twenty-three hours, while night owls may default to twenty-five or twenty-six.* To get up or to try to sleep on schedule when your circadian rhythm is running faster or slower than twenty-four hours was to put yourself out of synchrony with the rhythms of the base. But to sleep as you pleased would cause havoc to base routine, and upset the delicate harmony of its little society – there were just fourteen of us for the ten months the base was isolated. My role as the doctor was to look after the well-being of those on base, but also to investigate whether supplementing the dim fluorescent lighting on base with additional light boxes could keep everyone's body clocks to time, alternating white light with blue-enriched as the winter progressed.

Circadian rhythms influence more than just our waking and sleeping – they govern body temperature, blood pressure and aspects of our bodies from the biochemical level right up to the psychological. Light is the best stimulus to mould our sense of time, but exercise after waking can help, as can rigid mealtimes (the liver has a distinct body clock calibrated to customary mealtimes, just as the brain's clock is timed to sleep cycles). The pineal gland gets its knowledge about the seasons, and ambient light conditions, via 'ganglion cells' arising within the intricate weave of the retina. These neurons are a 'third eye', keeping the body aware of the passage of night and day in an entirely unconscious way, and they respond better to light at the blue end of the spectrum.†

The temperature outside reached the fifties below zero, but every 'afternoon' I would go skiing on a marked track around the three-kilometre perimeter of the base. I'd ski by moonlight if the moon could be seen, or starlight when it

---

* There are identifiable genes which code for these traits, and 'clock genes' can predict whether you are by habit early or late to bed.
† There are even people who are 'cortically blind', in the sense that they have no conscious perception of light, but this 'third eye' continues to keep the body clock running strictly to time.

could not. Sometimes I'd ski by the light of auroras. Gathering light into my eyes at the same time each day, I hoped to convince my brain that there was still a shape to the day.

THE SIMPLEST and most archaic organisms on earth, blue-green algae, have circadian rhythms: during daylight, special proteins gather like parasols over their DNA to prevent damage by the sun's radiation (in darkness those proteins move away to let DNA do its work). It's likely that the earliest organisms in the primordial ocean worked to a shorter rhythm than we're used to today, just twenty-two hours, because the earth was spinning faster when they first evolved. There was no ozone layer then, making it even more crucial that DNA be protected against the harsh, unfiltered sunlight. Many of the genes that govern our body's sense of time look as if they have evolved from primitive proteins involved in this ancient cycle of protecting and repairing DNA.

Many of our own cells – not just in the pineal gland or the liver – have what's called a 'molecular oscillator', showing a twenty-four-hour pattern to the genes they express, and varying throughout the day in terms of their electrical activity. At the molecular level the body is chemistry, and as a general rule chemical reactions go faster in the heat and slower in the cold. But body clock genes and the proteins they express can keep to time irrespective of background temperature – something of critical importance to insects, plants and other organisms that have no temperature control.

Jetlag exists because our bodies have a brake that slows adjustment whenever we move into a new rhythm of darkness and light. It's a form of resistance to change: the body shifts cautiously into the new rhythm, and it is that caution that prevents our rapid adjustment to a new ambient time zone. If body clocks were able to reset quickly and easily our ancestors might have been thrown out of kilter by a full moon, or whenever they enjoyed a late night around their Palaeolithic fires. But our body clocks have to be able to shift – without that malleability we could never have moved from the tropics to the temperate and polar latitudes as a species, where there are rapid swings in sunrise and sunset times around each equinox. Adaptability of the body's sense of time made it possible for humanity to move across immense distances of latitude, just as today it facilitates the jet-age shifts in longitude.

A few years ago, a group of cell biologists in Oxford found the cause for this 'brake' on adjustment to jetlag: when light shines on the ganglion cells within our retinas. But then another protein kicks in, switching those genes off again almost as soon as they're active. Adjustment to the new rhythm is delayed until the pressure of light exposure, day after day, becomes irrepressible. The researchers created transgenic mice without this molecular brake; the new mice adapted to an artificially induced jetlag of six hours within just a day or two, raising their hopes that one day there could be a drug that could cure jetlag, or help shift workers adjust to switching between night and day shifts.

IT'S MORE THAN A DECADE since I practised medicine in Antarctica, but I still meet with circadian problems in clinic. The rhythms of our bodies are often discordant with the rhythms of our communities and our working lives; people in the West spend on average an hour less a day out in natural light than they did twenty years ago, and screen time has burgeoned over the same period, cramming our brains with its blue-enriched light. Shift-working is endemic – particularly in healthcare – and to work rapidly alternating shifts is to condemn yourself to perpetual jetlag. Shift-working is known to lead to poorer concentration, as well as obesity – you get hungrier when your sleep is mistimed, crave more carbohydrate, and a sluggish, out-of-kilter metabolism exacerbates and accelerates diabetes and heart disease.

When the clocks change for winter, for many it's as if a door is gradually closing, or a curtain is being drawn across their mood and ability to concentrate. 'Winter blues' is one name for it, 'Seasonal Affective Disorder' another. Herman Melville described it in *Moby Dick*: 'Whenever I find myself growing grim about the mouth; whenever it is a damp, drizzling November in my soul …' To get away from winter blues Melville's narrator Ishmael took off to the South Seas, but most of us don't have that opportunity – we have to find a way to make our peace with the winter.

It can feel as much of a struggle to keep one's body clock running to time through a Scottish winter as it did through an Antarctic one. The research I conducted in Antarctica showed that the sky-blue light boxes offered a slight improvement in the quality of sleep, but didn't help any of our small group stay more closely to the twenty-four-hour clock. The best ways to beat winter blues, keep the body clock to time, as well as get over jetlag, remain the same wherever you are in the world: stick to a routine, eat well-spaced healthy meals, get daily exercise and, crucially, get as much light through the day as possible – natural light from the sky is usually many factors of magnitude brighter than artificial light. When I remember my time in Antarctica, skiing day after day beneath heavens as wide and dark as a dilated pupil, I was grateful for the spectacle of meteors and auroras, the phases of the moon and the ceaseless turning of the stars. My eyes, as organs of light, granted visions of great beauty there, but I appreciate them too, now, as organs of time.

17

Bonesetting: An Algebra of Healing

The treatment of a fracture is not difficult, and is almost any practitioner's job.

Hippocrates, *Fractures*

A YEAR AFTER FINISHING the job in Antarctica I flew out to West Africa to learn about the work of my friend Stephen, a paediatrician. He was carrying out some research on malnutrition, and running a back-country clinic near the Gambia's border with Senegal. The clinic lay to one side of a small village community and did basic, vital work as well as research: minor injuries, treatment of infections, pregnancy care, nutritional advice. There were no X-ray facilities and few drugs. Every morning as I ate breakfast I'd watch a queue lengthen from the clinic's front door along a shaded walkway and out into the surrounding trees. I had little experience of rural tropical medicine then, but hoped to learn.

It was April, the hottest month of the year, and the temperature climbed over 40°C. In the hottest part of the day it was impossible to work: I'd lie still in a hammock strung between two trees. The wind that came scorching out of the Sahara was like a furnace blast, warming the skin rather than cooling it. Within a year my skin had passed through a hundred degrees of heat – from the fifties below zero in Antarctica to the forties above. Vultures sat panting in the dust, wings outstretched to cool themselves, the way I'd seen penguins do when Antarctic temperatures approached the melting point of ice.

The sun fell so swiftly that there was little sense of an evening, but when the day's clinical work was done, and the temperature became more bearable, I'd take a walk through the village. Though at times it felt remote – there was no phone signal after 5 p.m., and the internet connection was vestigial – there were hints of the wider world. One of the village's earthen huts housed a bakery: when flour arrived from the coast you'd see smoke from its chimney, and know that there'd be French baguettes on sale. There was a small shop run by a Mauritanian pedlar, who sold lanterns and buckets made in China. Those goods were imported by Lebanese merchants who'd been settled for a century on the Atlantic coast. As he worked, the pedlar listened to the BBC World Service in Arabic.

If there was time I'd continue on towards the river, beneath a spreading mango tree, down an avenue of baobabs and through thickets of man-high yellow reeds. Beyond the reeds there were squared ridges of dry-baked soil – rice paddies in the wet season – then some mudflats and, in the distance, the brown slick of the river. I'd been brought up with the reliable rivers of northern Europe, but this was something altogether different: briny and unpredictable, an oily wallow of mud, fed by the fickle rains of the Saharan fringe. Lungfish flopped into holes at my approach, breathing heavily. It seemed a land where categories were unstable, and the unexpected was routine.

'GEOMETRY' MEANS 'measurement of the earth', and as a science it has its origins in ancient Egypt. It was used to calculate the land available for agriculture as the water level rose and fell in the fertile Nile delta. One of its foundational texts is Euclid's *Elements*, written in Alexandria around 300 BCE – said to be the most influential textbook ever written, second only to the Bible in terms of the number of editions that have been printed. It starts with defining terms ('a line is a breadthless length', 'a boundary is an extremity of any thing') and goes on to postulate various axioms ('the whole is greater than the part', 'all right angles are equal to one another'). From these definitions and axioms it constructs a whole mathematical world, then tames it. Proofs tumble from its pages. One of the most famous of its proofs shows how the two basal angles of an isosceles triangle must always be equal. In the Middle Ages, scholars gave this proof the name 'Bridge of Asses', because students who struggled with it were unlikely to progress.

At school I always enjoyed mathematics; I liked its absence of words, the way it encouraged visualisation of the infinite, and its reliable delivery of neat conclusions – at my level at least. There was pleasure in mastering each new technique: now the circumference of a circle, now the length of a hypotenuse, now the gradient of a curve. Calculus was particularly satisfying – a kind of arithmetical magic. That a string of letters and numbers could be transformed into a sweeping parabola was an unexpected delight.

I learned that one inventor of calculus was Isaac Newton and that for him transformation was a universal, elemental process: everything in flux that could be measured and portrayed in algebraic form he termed a 'fluent'. His mathematics summoned a world of ceaselessly changing rivers of numbers. He invented calculus to describe the rate of change of each fluent, which he called 'fluxion'.

The word *algebra* is Arabic, *al-jabr*, which means 'bonesetting'. Although there are hints of algebra in ancient Greek texts such as Euclid's *Elements*, and even in the writings of the Greek physician Galen, the algebra that we know today was invented in ninth-century Baghdad. The mathematics of algebra was named for bonesetting because it pulls apart two sides of an equation, balances them, then resolves them to find solutions – just as a broken bone could be pulled apart in traction and then made to heal. In southern Spain, thanks to the legacy of the Arabs, bonesetters and barber surgeons were known until modern times as *algebristas*.

One of the great reassurances of mathematics is that equations work out the same every time. The human way of healing doesn't fit well into the ethereal perfection of mathematical formulae: it's different for every individual, and every injury. Mathematics can probe transcendent mysteries such as prime numbers reaching into infinity, or the impossible calculation of negative square roots. The business of human healing is messier, though no less mysterious.

ONE AFTERNOON A BOY of eight was carried into the Gambian clinic having fallen ten feet from a mango tree and injured a leg. He was unable to walk and, sobbing with pain, wouldn't let anyone examine him. Stephen injected local anaesthetic into the groin at the top of his left leg to numb the thigh, which allowed the boy, eventually, to straighten his hips. His left leg looked shorter than it should have, and his left knee was turned out to one side – both signs suggesting his femur had been fractured. It was a life-threatening injury: femoral fractures can prove fatal either from blood loss within the leg or from pneumonias that set in with immobility. The best way to ease the pain of these fractures is to pull the leg out into traction on a frame called a Thomas splint, which restores the thigh to its normal length and brings the snapped ends of bone together.

Thomas splints are named for a Welsh surgeon called Hugh Owen Thomas, who came from a long line of Anglesey bonesetters – perhaps his 'innovation' was simply the adaptation of a family secret. I'd had two of these 'Thomas splints' in my clinic in Antarctica and never needed to use them. In the Gambia, where I really needed one, there were none available.

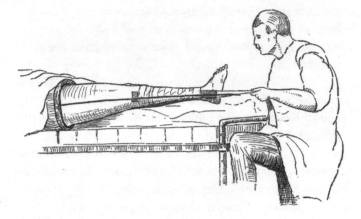

We wrapped the boy's leg in loose bandages and made a box with pieces of wood lined with crumpled tissue paper – he'd be more comfortable with the leg immobilised, but without the traction of the Thomas splint his leg still looked shorter than it should. The only way to assess his injury thoroughly would be to get an X-ray, which meant a four-hour journey, on dirt roads, to a clinic on the Atlantic coast.

The boy's father was a solemn old man, stately in his dirty white robe and skull cap. No, he said, the boy wouldn't go to the coast. He knew someone who had gone there with a fractured leg and had never returned. The boy would come home with him and they'd see a bonesetter in the village.

Some of the nurses began to get angry, accusing the father of child abuse. He was threatened with a call to the police. I tried to explain through interpreters that there was a chance the boy would be crippled, that his leg would shorten and tilt unless it was treated correctly. But with dignity the man simply gathered his boy in his arms and walked off through the trees.

FOR MANY CENTURIES algebra evolved in parallel with geometry, rather than integrated with it. They were thought of as mutually exclusive mathematical systems: geometry was the more distinguished elder cousin, representing the world in concrete terms that were discrete and universally applicable. Algebra was the newcomer, a slippery, Arab-inflected symbolism which, for many in the West, carried a hint of the occult (the philosopher Thomas Hobbes called it 'a scab of symbols').

It was Descartes, the philosopher of division between body and mind, who finally unified algebra with geometry. He showed how the two disciplines were part of the same cosmic continuum, that together they could resolve mathematical problems that had previously been insoluble. He plotted geometrical shapes on perpendicular axes that we still call 'Cartesian coordinates' in his honour, giving the letter 'x' to one axis, and 'y' to the other. He had devised a system of mapping shapes of infinite dimensions.

With his division of body and mind, Descartes broke the physical world into parts and processes, heralding the specialisation of science and medicine and unleashing a revolution in thought still reverberating today. And with his fusion of algebra with geometry he paved the way for calculus, for a mathematics of transformation to fit the churning, evolving world.

A WEEK AFTER THE INCIDENT with the boy and the broken leg I drove out with Kalilu, one of the clinic's nurses, to another village to deliver 'directly observed' tuberculosis therapy ('DOT'). Kalilu wore a neat Islamic beard with no moustache, and wore a black woollen skull cap. His spectacle frames were ornate and golden, and clipped to his nursing uniform he carried a mobile phone. He had a calm air of imperturbability, and told me that he hoped one day to study in the UK. On the drive he told me about the DOT initiative to ensure adequate treatment of TB, and to limit its spread. We roared away from the clinic into the loose, Sahel scrubland, beeping at donkeys and goats that strayed into our path. Baboons loped across the road ahead of us, green vervet monkeys swung up into the trees. There were no road signs, but termite mounds towered along each verge like snow poles. The track was not so much potholed as undulating; sometimes the earth looked scorched, but whether deliberately cleared for agriculture or accidentally ignited by a stray cigarette, Kalilu couldn't say. We drove past swamps, savannah and rubble-fields of volcanic rocks. The air felt gritty with Sahara-blown sand. The landscape was so beautiful that I didn't want the journey to end, but suddenly I saw tin and thatched roofs appear through the trees, announced by a tired UNICEF notice: 'Baby Friendly Community'.

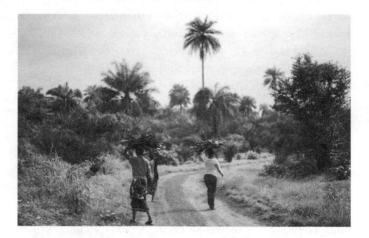

We slowed as we entered the village. Groups of men sat in the shade and waved to Kalilu as we passed. The women were all working: carrying wood, pounding flour. Children ran from the earthen-walled houses to follow the car, surrounding us as we emerged, shouting 'What-is-your-name-what-is-your-name.'

'Just say, "Tubab",' said Kalilu. 'It means "white man".'

He led me to an earthen-walled house with a corrugated steel door; an old woman sat in the shade outside. Beside her stood a naked boy aged two or three who gazed open-mouthed at my pale skin. We went in and called but there was no answer. Inside there were two rooms: one bare, its walls washed in white, a torn cloth mattress rolled up in one corner. The other room was empty but for a well-made double bed and, on it, a dirty throw. We walked back out, Kalilu calling for his patient. A crowd began to gather, then a young woman in an ankle-length sarong and matching headscarf stepped forward, laughing. She directed us back into the house: our patient had been sleeping under the dirty throw.

The man who emerged from beneath the throw was so thin that each joint and ligament, each vein and tendon, stood out as if he'd been flayed. He acknowledged his audience (spectators were crowding into the room), lit a cigarette stub, and with a groan pulled himself over to the edge of the bed. Kalilu poured the correct dose and combination of anti-tuberculous pills into a cup. No, the patient said, shaking his head. He wouldn't take them. There were too many, and they made him feel sick. 'See how thin he is,' muttered Kalilu to me, tut-tutting. 'He has refused a test for HIV.' More of the man's family began to appear, pushing through the onlookers, raising their voices and pointing. 'They are telling him not to be stupid,' Kalilu translated, 'they are telling him to take the medicine.' Village elders arrived, and gave more indignant advice. Most onlookers seemed amused, but their voices began to edge with impatience. Still the man sat calmly, smoking and shaking his head as the villagers remonstrated with him.

As with the boy with the broken leg, I knew that having treatment available for a particular medical problem didn't mean that I knew how to persuade a patient to accept it. And then there were the wider economics of his situation: in nineteenth-century Britain, before anti-TB treatments had been developed, death from the disease was directly linked to the sufferer's level of poverty. Even with effective drugs available, the link between poverty and TB deaths remains stubbornly robust. To treat the man's TB effectively, he had to be cured of his poverty and, as a doctor, I didn't have the first idea how to approach that.

I asked Kalilu what he was saying to the man. He said: 'I'm telling him the tubab doctor is ordering him to take the medicine.'

The man pointed up at me and said something – everyone laughed.

'What did he say?'

'"If the tubab wants me to take them, he can pay me",' Kalilu said.

Kalilu shook his head and laughed at the suggestion – though hidden within it was the tacit acknowledgement that money was as necessary as medicine in the cure of this disease. Resistance broke: the crowd looked on silently while one by one the man took the tablets, swigging them down with cola before falling back on the mattress and pulling the throw over his shoulders. The women drifted back to their work, the men to the shade, the children to their games.

IN THE FIRST PHASE of bone healing there's a flare of inflammation, with clotted blood forming around the broken ends, and the body's immune system provokes pain and swelling. The blood clot becomes a framework for tough, fibrous cells, and the lining of each bone (the 'periosteum') transforms into a tissue that can lay down new cartilage and bone. This new bone grows out in a bulbous mass from each end of the fracture, until they meet one another in the middle to form a bridge of 'fracture callus'. This process may take days with a small bone or weeks with a large one. How close the broken ends are to one another, and how well aligned, influences the speed of healing.

The new bone to be laid down is spongy and frail; over further weeks it is gradually replaced with layered, stronger, 'lamellar' bone. Lamellar bone is then remodelled by specialised cells that streamline the callus outline. Sometimes I see X-rays in which the fracture healing has been perfect – there's little sign on the image that there's been any injury at all. At other times lumpy irregularities and thickenings endure, and I'll be able to turn to a surprised patient and ask 'So when did you break your ribs?' Small bones, like the ones in the fingers, may be fully healed by three weeks. A bone like the femur may take twelve.

As I walked back to the car with Kalilu, I saw the boy of the week before, limping along after his friends. 'Look!' I said to Kalilu, pointing over to him. 'There's that boy with the femoral fracture. But those fractures take six weeks at least.'

Kalilu shrugged. 'Maybe the bonesetter worked some magic. Maybe you were wrong – the leg wasn't broken at all.'

We drove back into the bush, which seemed less beautiful on the return journey. Rather than admire the scenery I thought about the economics of health and how much about being a doctor I was yet to learn. Another day working in medicine, another Bridge of Asses I struggled to cross.

18

Menopause: Third Face of the Goddess

The menopause is probably the least glamorous topic imaginable; and this is interesting, because it is one of the very few topics to which cling some shreds and remnants of taboo.

Ursula K. Le Guin, 'The Space Crone'

EDINBURGH'S MENOPAUSE CLINIC is held in the Chalmers Sexual Health Centre – an old Victorian hospital first opened in 1864 at the bequest of a master plumber. George Chalmers specified in his will that he wanted a 'New Infirmary or Sick and Hurt Hospital, or by whatever name it may be Designed'. The lower two wards were for the destitute, the upper two wards for those who could pay three shillings a day. 'In 1887 a small apartment for nurses was opened,' says the official history; 'It lay between the wine cellar and the mortuary.'

Sometime in the 1950s the building amalgamated with the nearby Hospital for the Diseases of Women, and through slow metamorphosis shed its lying-in wards. In 2011 it was refurbished as the city's sexual health centre, with a mixed bag of specialisms: venereal diseases, contraception, menopause, as well as the gender identity clinic. Queues lengthen outside every morning for the drop-in service. Jokers or prudes have prised the word 'Sexual' from its sandstone wall.

Most of the sexual health clinics I've worked in have a jaunty, informal atmosphere; their patients are fairly young, the diseases for the most part are treatable (now that even HIV is kept in abeyance), and the staff have a gentle irreverence that lends itself to a good working environment. All doctors hear stories that must remain private, but sexual health physicians hear more than their share.

When I went to learn more about the work of the menopause clinic I started in the coffee room, where students, trainees and consultants were all laughing together over stories from a staff night out. I was there to sit in with Ailsa Gebbie, a consultant gynaecologist and the senior clinician at the menopause clinic. Ailsa had been one of my tutors at medical school twenty years earlier – energetic and enthusiastic, with short blonde hair and a crisp, careful manner of speaking. She's a former vice-president of the UK's Faculty of Sexual and Reproductive Healthcare.

Few women come to my clinic for advice about the menopause – I'm a forty-something man, and they generally prefer to consult a female colleague. But every so often someone going through what still gets called 'the change of life' asks me about hot flushes, insomnia, skin changes or mood swings. Oestrogen slows over years rather than months, making the name 'menopause' sound more abrupt than the reality. Meno-*pause* also suggests something temporary, even trivial. Symptoms of the menopause may be transient and often mild, but the phase it gives onto is enduring and hardly trivial. Menopause isn't a disease, or a deficiency, or even a constellation of symptoms, but a natural consequence of having lived for four or five decades as a woman. All women see a dramatic drop in oestrogen levels around menopause, but only about one in fifty men sees a comparable drop in testosterone levels at the same age. Around a third of women suffer enough from it to want to see a doctor, ranging from those exhausted, distressed and depressed by their symptoms, to those who'd just like to attenuate their hot flushes. As a man, I see too few women in this situation to keep up with the latest advice, but too many to refer them all to a colleague. So I went to sit in with Ailsa to see what I could learn.

BEFORE 'MENOPAUSE' WAS COINED a little over a century ago, the clunky Greek term 'climacteric' was used more widely. The word means a step on a ladder – a phase to be transcended or surpassed – but 'climacteric' has been made to bear a heavy burden of meanings: a climax to life, a critical period, a storm successfully weathered. For much of its history it applied to men as much as it did to women, though men's 'climacterical year' was traditionally thought to be the sixty-third – long after the forty-ninth year suggested for women. Pre-modern medicine was preoccupied with numerology and had an obsession with factors of seven that goes back at least to Solon of Athens, who in around 600 BCE wrote a long poem about the way that human life is divided into ages of seven years, each initiated by a rite of passage and occasioning a change in role. But the association with sevens is more ancient still: the Babylonians noticed seven celestial bodies (Sun, Moon, Mercury, Venus, Mars, Jupiter, Saturn) and built seven levels to their ziggurats; Greek language took seven vowels, and defined seven wonders of the world.

There are three columns of discussion in the *Oxford English Dictionary* devoted to 'climacteric', and only one entry refers specifically to the menopause: 'Applied to that period in life (usually between the ages of 45 and 60) when the vital forces begin to decline (in women coinciding with the period of "change of life").' For the term 'climacteric disease' it offers: 'a disease of unknown cause which often occurs at an advanced stage of life, characterized by loss of flesh and strength, sleeplessness, etc.'

Of the four hundred or so editors and contributors who worked on the *OED*, about seventy were women. The 'C' section that includes 'climacteric' was overseen by four.* But the exclusion of women's voices from much of literature's history means that every original source for 'climacteric' they recorded, written between 1590 and 1879, was written by a man.

The historian Louise Foxcroft, in her book *Hot Flushes, Cold Science: A History of the Menopause*, summarises the historical male take on menopause by quoting the sixteenth-century physician Giovanni Marinello: 'as soon as the periods stop, pains arise ... the disorderly uterus rises or descends all the time, or commits other actions difficult to endure.' Foxcroft warns against thinking of the climacteric as a purely female phenomenon: 'Men have hormones too,' she observes, 'and arguably, a menopause, if we think of it as a transitional phase which is part of the ageing process.'

The historian of medicine Roy Porter warned about the domination of masculine perspectives, particularly with respect to discussions of women's bodies. Porter's opinion was that menopausal problems, when they present at all, are overblown and the result of a male orientated profession's tendency to medicalise whatever it doesn't understand. He reported that in many traditional societies there's an absence of subjective problems with menopause – that, on the contrary, menopause was something that women celebrated, because it marked release from a part of their lives that was often 'burdensome and dangerous' (bearing children), as well as stigmatising (menstruation being viewed as polluting). Cross-cultural studies of women around the climacteric bear up Porter's analysis: Finnish, Mayan, North African, Rajput, Chinese and Japanese women

---

* Miss J. E. A. Brown, Miss Edith Thompson, Miss E. R. Steane and Mrs W. Noel Woods.

have all been found by researchers to suffer fewer physical or 'somatic' menopausal symptoms than, for example, American women. A 1980s study by Nancy Datan examined five ethnic groups in Israel – Muslim Arabs as well as Jews from North Africa, Persia, Turkey and central Europe – and found that each welcomed the menopause as a liberation. As human beings, wrote Datan, we are all in different states of transition, 'immigrants in middle and old age to a changing world for which we are not prepared'. She concluded that each ethnic group had traditions which helped women adopt new and liberating roles in middle age, and that every culture finds ways of infusing life with love and with meaningful work.

In the twentieth century, medicine began characterising menopause as a deficiency disease, treatable by Hormonal Replacement Therapy (HRT) – first launched in 1942. Twenty years later, HRT was applauded into the pharmacies and stock exchanges of the world by a New York gynaecologist called Robert A. Wilson, whose book *Feminine Forever* suggested that women should consider HRT in their thirties or risk crumbling bones and collapsing libidos. Wilson called women who'd been through the menopause 'castrates'.

In the final years of the medicalising twentieth century, 27,000 post-menopausal women took part in the 'Women's Health Initiative' study, the results of which implied that women taking HRT had a slightly higher risk of strokes and breast cancer than those who didn't. Then in 2003 a far larger study, appropriately named 'The Million Women Study', suggested that taking HRT as much as *doubled* the risk of breast cancer, though the absolute numbers remained small. Headline writers are prone to prioritise relative risk over absolute risk: an increase of 1 in 100,000 adverse events to 2 in 100,000 is an almost insignificant change, but a headline may still scream that risk has 'doubled'. The effect was immediate – between 2002 and 2006 HRT prescription in the UK dropped by two-thirds. These trials were shown to be fundamentally flawed, using the same doses of hormones in women aged forty who'd gone into an early menopause as they did in women aged seventy who'd had a natural menopause twenty years earlier.

HRT remains controversial. Before going along to the menopause clinic I asked Iona Heath, former president of the Royal College of General Practitioners and for thirty-five years a practising GP, for her perspective on the merits and hazards of HRT. 'When I meet a menopausal woman in clinic who wants help with her symptoms I tell her there are two ways to look at the HRT controversy,' she told me. 'The first is that HRT is a male-dominated conspiracy to medicalise a normal, natural process.'

'And the second?'

'That the scare stories about HRT are a male-dominated conspiracy to stop women getting the hormone supplements they need. The way they respond would tell me which way they wanted to go.'

WHEN CHALMERS'S HOSPITAL first opened in the 1860s a girl born in its wards would have had a life expectancy of about forty-one. By the late 1880s, when nurses' quarters were opened by the mortuary, that life expectancy had risen to just forty-five. These figures were so low because of the terrible frequency with which women (and babies) died in childbirth. The majority of female children didn't live to reach the menopause, and those who did were relatively rare – resilient survivors.

Ailsa led me from the coffee room along a whitewashed mezzanine corridor. The refurbishment had given this third phase of Chalmers' hospital a new and repurposed life – it had gained a glass roof, they had rebuilt some walls, and natural light fell in shafts past a space where once there had been gynaecology and obstetric wards. 'Will the clinic today be all new patients?' I asked Ailsa.

'A mixture – some of these women I review after a few months if they are trying out different treatments. Some of them will be new to me – referred in because their usual doctor can't get their symptoms under control.'

'Will they all have been on HRT already?'

'Most of them – though there are still a few GPs who are anxious about prescribing, particularly if there are complications – a family history of cancer, thrombosis, strokes.'

I sat beside Ailsa while she conducted her clinic, meeting her patients, discussing with her how I'd manage each in my own clinic, taking notes for my own future practice. Many of the women clearly knew and trusted Ailsa; there were discussions about hot flushes, sexual problems, urinary infections, incontinence, osteoporosis, libido, crashing mood swings. Some women had gone into the menopause gradually, others in abrupt consequence of treatments for breast or ovarian cancer. 'In someone suffering severe hot flushes from cancer treatment there's good evidence for cognitive behavioural therapy rather than HRT,' Ailsa told me. 'Some kinds of counselling can be as good as HRT, perhaps even better, at helping people adjust to mood and sleep problems. And without the risks.'

'And what do you tell people about those risks?' I asked her.

'I show them a table that lays them out.' She opened the UK bible of prescribing – the *British National Formulary* – to a page listing the statistical risks. 'It shows how cancer and thrombosis risks begin to rise a little after ten years of continuous treatment. But those risks remain small.' For women in their fifties who've taken HRT for over ten years, breast cancer rates rose from about 2 per cent to just over 4 per cent. For women in their sixties the incidence rose from 3 per cent to just under 7 per cent.

'So it doubles, more or less,' I said.

'But it's still small. When people know the actual risk at a population level, rather than the relative risk, and their symptoms are intolerable, they often prefer the HRT. And generally You have to weigh up the risks and benefits, and remember that it's beyond sixty years of age that the cancer and thrombosis rates begin to rise.'

I saw Ailsa prescribe antidepressants rather than hormones on occasion, and I asked her whether she thought that meant mood changes and sleep problems around the menopause were related to depression and anxiety. 'Not always,' she said, 'but small doses of antidepressants can be helpful. No two women are the same.' Sex hormones maintain bone strength, so with menopause can come a thinning and weakening of bones. Ailsa prescribed medications to slow that process, and she also encouraged a couple of the women to smoke less and exercise more (smoking weakens bones, and exercise strengthens them). While most of the HRT I've ever prescribed has come in tablets, Ailsa suggested alternatives. 'Skin patches and gels that you rub into the skin of your thigh or buttock can be very useful – lower doses, fewer risks. If the only issue is that the skin of the vagina is getting thin and dry, or the bladder is prone to infection, you can prescribe a vaginal cream or pessary, or even a ring that women can put in the vagina and take out themselves, giving the oestrogen directly where you need it in a very low dose.'

Perhaps it's not possible, as a doctor, to make an objective judgement, but, in sitting for an afternoon with Ailsa, I didn't see any evidence of an overbearing medical establishment attempting to convince women they were suffering a deficiency disease. I saw women with anxiety, unbearable hot flushes, sexual difficulties and insomnia, some of which may have been brought on by a slowdown of body oestrogen, receive careful, balanced and often life-changing advice.

'AT MENOPAUSE as never before, a woman comes face to face with her own mortality,' wrote Germaine Greer in *The Change*. 'When a fifty-year-old woman says to herself, "Now is the best time of all", she means it all the more because she knows it is not forever.' The feminist psychologist Carol Gilligan noticed that the climacteric, as one of life's most significant transitions, can occasion a kind of mourning that 'can give way to the melancholia of self-depreciation and despair'. But there are other, more positive perspectives on menopause.

In 1976, the American novelist Ursula Le Guin wrote an essay both panoramic in scope and beautifully concise, reflecting on her own arrival at the change. I can't speak with authority or experience on the menopause, but Le Guin can, and I've recommended her essay to patients. She argues in the essay that the traditional division of women's lives into the triple phases of 'maidenhood', 'maturity' and 'crone' gave life a meaning and trajectory that was more than just a physical evolution – it was about social shifts in being. Le Guin views the late twentieth century as undervaluing virginity, with children acting more and more as young adults, while post-menopausal women are encouraged to take hormones to perpetuate youth. It is as if 'the Triple Goddess has only one face: Marilyn Monroe's, maybe,' she wrote.

Her proposal was that women become more comfortable with accepting the third stage in their lives, valuing it for something uniquely feminine, and offering liberating opportunities: 'The woman who is willing to make that change must become pregnant with herself, at last. She must bear herself, her third self, her old age, with travail and alone.' Unlike the births she'd laboured with her own children, no male obstetrician would stand over this new transition, or suture up her lacerations. 'Anyhow it seems a pity to have a built-in rite of passage and to dodge it, evade it, and pretend nothing has changed. That is to dodge and evade one's womanhood, to pretend one's like a man.'

Many readers know Le Guin through her body of science fiction and fantasy novels, and she concludes her essay with a sci-fi thought experiment: imagine some aliens asked to take 'an exemplary person' back to their planet Altair to teach them something of the nature of humanity. Le Guin wouldn't pick a young cosmonaut, or a male scientist, or even a statesman like Henry Kissinger. Neither would she pick one of the many young women who'd volunteer, 'some out of magnanimity and intellectual courage, others out of a profound conviction that Altair couldn't possibly be any worse for a woman than Earth is.' Instead she'd pick a woman over sixty – wise, patient, witty and shrewd – who'd worked hard all her life, given birth and raised her own children. She'll be too modest to volunteer, says Le Guin, but we should insist, because as a woman in the third stage of life she 'has experienced, accepted, and acted the entire human condition – the essential quality of which is Change.'

19

Castration: Hope, Love and Sacrifice

We defend ourselves not against castration anxiety but against death, a far more absolute castration.

Ernest Becker, *The Denial of Death*

THE UNIVERSITY LIBRARY at my medical school was shared with students of Veterinary Medicine. Sometimes I'd find myself at a desk opposite one of the vet students; we'd glance at one another's textbooks with curiosity, occasionally open at the same subjects – haematology, say, or orthopaedic surgery. It was reassuring to see how much common ground there was between medicine for humans and medicine for animals.

One day I was revising prostate cancer: the appearance of its malignant cells under a microscope, the stages of its spread, the radiotherapy, brachytherapy (embedding of radioactive pellets into the tumour), and standard chemotherapies used to treat it. In health, the prostate gland stores semen and mature sperm; it has strong muscular walls that squeeze during ejaculation. Exposure to a lifetime of testosterone increases the growth of the gland as well as its susceptibility to cancers. Many treatments for prostate cancer work by blocking testosterone's generation within the testicles – with no testosterone, the growth of the tumour slows.

'All that for prostate cancer?' asked one of the vet students, glancing over at my notes.

'Sure,' I said; 'what do you guys do to treat it?'

'One word,' he laughed, 'castration!'

As a boy I'd see farmers castrating spring lambs in the fields near my home. They'd take a tiny rubber 'O', the diameter of its hole almost as wide as the rubber was thick, and with a pair of special pliers spring it over the lamb's scrotum. The rubber squeezed off the blood supply to the testes, and a few weeks later they'd drop off. The first time I saw farmers gelding lambs I asked one of them, 'Doesn't it hurt?'

He shrugged. 'It's better this than the old way,' he replied. 'A century ago, shepherds used their teeth.' After an afternoon spent gelding, the men's beards would be clotted with blood.

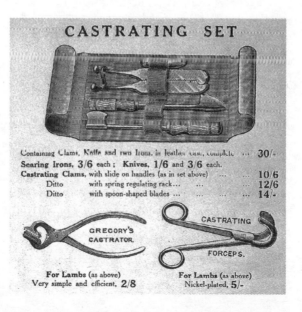

CASTRATING SET

Containing Clams, Knife and two Irons, in leather case, complete ... 30/-
Searing Irons, 3/6 each ; Knives, 1/6 and 3/6 each.
Castrating Clams, with slide on handles (as in set above) 10/6
   Ditto   with spring regulating rack... ... ... 12/6
   Ditto   with spoon-shaped blades 14/-

GREGORY'S CASTRATOR.

CASTRATING

FORCEPS.

For Lambs (as above)
Very simple and efficient, 2/8

For Lambs (as above)
Nickel-plated, 5/-

Gelding animals takes testosterone out of their development, making them less aggressive and more biddable, but also bigger (sex hormones accelerate the closure of the growth plates of bones, so without testosterone, animals' bones grow longer before fusing). Low testosterone levels also encourage the accumulation of fat. You can leave castrated animals grazing alongside females without fear they'll reproduce. Agricultural societies have used it since long before written records: castrated oxen take a yoke more easily, and will pull a plough with less whipping. Castrated dogs are simpler to train, and will more readily round up the castrated sheep put out to fatten in the fields. Early Assyrian and Chinese civilisations transposed this knowledge to humans: boys born in poverty would be castrated and sent to work under the yoke of the state in the imperial household. (In China, both penis and testicles were removed – these 'three treasures' were pickled in a jar, brought out for special occasions, and buried with the eunuch.) Eunuchs were often taller, sometimes stronger than average, and were frequently employed as the core of an imperial guard. They could work in the imperial harem without fear that they'd cuckold the emperor.

When Alexander the Great conquered Persia he was struck by the utility of such eunuch slaves, and adopted the custom – eunuchs were also considered sexually desirable. The Romans copied it from the Greeks: the emperor Nero had a eunuch called Sporus (whom he dressed as a woman, and married) and the emperor Domitian had a favourite eunuch called Earinus. There's usually an element of voyeurism in the Roman accounts, a curiosity about ambiguous gender and genitalia that's still visible in media coverage of the phenomenon today. Eunuchs were high-class slaves, the most expensive in the market; in losing testicles they were believed to have lost family loyalty and to have become faithful only to their masters and to the empire.

Around the time that Christianity began to spread into

the Roman Empire there was already a cult of a eunuch god called Attis, who was celebrated in springtime and believed to have died then been resurrected after three days. His priests committed self-castration in honour of a fertility goddess, and they did it on the hill in Rome where Vatican City sits now. The practice survived the Christianisation of the Roman Empire: one of the early church fathers, Origen, is famous for committing self-castration. Castration continued in Byzantium (where gelded boys were trained as choristers) and into the twentieth-century Russian Orthodox church, where the *skoptsy* sect encouraged self-castration as late as the 1920s. St Paul's advice that women should keep quiet in church was taken to its logical conclusion during the Italian Renaissance: God's glory was sung in soprano by castrated men from the mid-1500s. The Jesuit Tommaso Tamburini, active in the early seventeenth century, sanctioned castration only 'provided there is no mortal danger to life and that it is not done without the boy's consent'. How much choice they had in the matter is hard to assess, though reports throughout the seventeenth and eighteenth centuries describe boys 'pleading' for the honour of being castrated, to bring both prestige and financial security to their families. The complex, high-pitched melodies for which castrati were most in demand by the Vatican were those sung around Easter week – the same time of year that the priests of Attis celebrated castration.

The Vatican didn't ban the castration of boys for its choirs until the late nineteenth century, and the last castrato of the Sistine Chapel, Alessandro Moreschi, died in 1922. But twenty years before he died, with his voice already fading in quality, he made a series of recordings for the 'Gramophone and Typewriter Company' that would become 'His Master's Voice' or HMV. You can find the recordings online, Moreschi's voice a wavering, ghostly soprano that makes every song an elegy.

THE COMEDIAN BILLY CONNOLLY once joked that he'd reached an age when doctors had become uninterested in his balls, and had begun showing greater interest in his rectum. The median age for testicular cancer is around thirty-four, for prostate cancer it's nearer seventy-two. To have your prostate gland checked manually you have to lie on one side, knees pulled up to your chest, while a doctor puts a gloved finger in through your anus – the size and consistency of the prostate can be assessed through the thin bowel wall.

Prostate cancer is common: among my local patient population of almost four thousand, there are several new diagnoses a year. Alex Sinclair was one of them: a sixty-two-year-old builder, muscular and stoical, bald, with a beard so dense and black it was as if the lower half of his face was eclipsed. He told me he was divorced, and hinted at a dynamic sex life; his children had long ago grown up and moved away. He came to clinic wearing his overalls. 'I used to get up once or twice a night to pee,' he told me, 'but now it can be five or six times. I wake up exhausted.' There were times he found himself standing at the toilet for a full minute before urine began to trickle out. 'I prefer not to see doctors,' he said. 'But I couldn't put it off any more.'

We worked through a questionnaire called the 'International Prostate Symptom Score' which asks for a rating of one to five across a series of questions, from how often you have had the sense that you haven't emptied your bladder, to how often you have to strain to initiate urine flow: Alex scored an impressive twenty-two. I took a blood sample from his arm, to examine levels of a substance specific to the prostate – this 'PSA test' varies broadly with prostate size, and can on occasion flag up cancer. I asked if I could do a rectal examination up on the couch. 'I've heard about these,' he said with resignation, standing up to unzip his overalls; 'if you must.'

Alex's prostate was huge, jutting back from its position

under the bladder and indenting his rectum. On one side of the crease down the middle of the gland I felt a firmer, discrete lump, like a pebble lodged in tarmac.

'Well, that's why you've been struggling,' I told him; 'your prostate is so large, urine can hardly squeeze through it.' Alex stood up and started pulling up his overalls. 'I'd like you to see one of the specialists,' I added, then caught and held his eye. 'They'll want to check tiny pieces of the gland under a microscope.'

His actions slowed as he took in this information. Then he asked carefully: 'How do they get the pieces out?'

'They'll pass a very fine needle in through your anus, and through the bowel wall.' I was hoping to reassure, but wondered if perhaps I was making his anxiety worse. 'Your prostate gets bigger the longer it's been exposed to the testosterone in your body – so the longer you've lived, the bigger your prostate grows. You're not alone – it's quite common to start getting problems around your age.'

'Is it the same thing as cancer?' he asked, pulling up his zip and reaching for his hat.

I waited a couple of moments, until again his gaze swung back towards me. 'Just as every man's prostate grows the longer he's lived, they say every man gets prostate cancer if he lives long enough. But in most men it grows slowly, and never causes bother.'

'How will I know if it's going to cause bother with me?'

THROUGH THE 1980S, an editor at *The New York Times* called Anatole Broyard wrote a series of short, brilliant essays about being diagnosed and treated for prostate cancer. The essays were collected and published by his widow following his death from the illness. Broyard had for many years been a literary critic, and he brought to the essays an immense breadth of reference, humour, a ferocious intellect, and prose as luminous as an arc light. 'What goes through your mind when you're lying, full of nuclear dye, under a huge machine that scans all your bones for evidence of treason?', he wrote of one scan, undertaken to see if cancer had infiltrated his skeleton; 'There's a horror-movie appeal to this machine: Beneath it you become the Frankenstein monster exposed to the electric storm.'

Broyard experienced his own diagnosis as a storm of anxiety and fear, but also, paradoxically, a liberation – life became as colourful as a 'paisley shawl draped over a grand piano'. As a critic he turned to books to help him come to terms with his cancer, but complained that too many memoirs were humourless, over-respectful, and soaked in Romanticism, 'so pious they sound as if they were written on tip-toe'. He admitted that a part of him felt exalted by the diagnosis, as if in hearing some of the worst news anyone can hear – a diagnosis of terminal illness – he'd been granted a great blessing by the universe. There was an element of gratitude for some aspects of his illness: it had given him a deeper and more intimate appreciation of the glory of being alive, as well as licence to give in to a long-suppressed desire to be more impulsive.

In an essay called 'The Patient Examines the Doctor', he spells out the kind of physician he'd prefer – someone with a 'furious desire to oppose himself to fate ... intense enough or wilful enough to prevail over something powerful and demonic like illness'. Broyard often felt that he had to put on a stoical front for his friends, who'd congratulate him on his bravery, but knew that a good doctor should see through the bravado and recognise his loneliness, even act as a guide through the inferno of cancer therapy. He didn't want a doctor that relied on bluster, or phoney confidence tricks. His ideal doctor would be schooled in poetry, or be at least familiar with the possibilities of metaphor:

> I would like a doctor who is not only a talented physician, but a bit of a metaphysician, too. Someone who can treat body and soul .... To get to my body,

my doctor has to get to my character. He has to go through my soul. He doesn't only have to go through my anus.

Broyard refused the physical castration his first surgeon offered ('My urologist, who is quite famous, wanted to cut off my testicles, but I felt that this would be losing the battle right at the beginning'); but he accepted that most treatments for his prostate cancer might make him impotent, or affect his libido. He advised against thinking of sex as physical, rather than an intimate extension of the imagination, and accepted the diminution of his sex life as a reasonable bargain in the hope of gaining more years of life. 'In my own case,' he wrote, 'after a brush with death, I feel that just to be alive is a permanent orgasm.'

THE UROLOGISTS CONFIRMED IT: Alex had prostate cancer. What's more it had spread, and so removing his prostate gland to eliminate the tumour wasn't an option. The first step to improving his quality of life was to widen the urinary passage through the prostate, or 'bore it out' as Alex put it (builders have a useful store of analogies when thinking about the body and its failings). I had assisted in these operations as a junior doctor: a patient was laid anaesthetised on their back, legs in stirrups, while a narrow instrument with a camera inside it was advanced down through the penis and into the bladder. It was always an amazement to watch the procedure, the camera exploring an unseen, barely credible world of pink tunnels and embankments, delicately veined and whorled with contours. Once into the prostate a wire loop emerged from the instrument, which, when heated up by an electric current, could simultaneously peel away and cauterise the tissue that had been blocking the urine's flow. It took a few days for the bleeding to settle down – days in which Alex had to stay in hospital with a wide-bore catheter draining the bladder. Following the procedure Alex's urine was flowing, but his cancer was too far advanced to be eliminated. I started him on injections to shut down the production of testosterone in the testes, as well as hormone blockers. Plans were made for radiotherapy at the local hospital.

I reviewed him a couple of weeks after the first injection. His interest in sex had collapsed, his skin felt hot and dry, his urine heavy and stinging. 'I've never been much of a worrier,' he told me, 'but I'm getting uptight about everything these days. And I can't watch a film without blubbing like a baby.' He wanted to continue working, but found his muscles ached after even minimal exercise, and he was losing much of his strength. These were all symptoms that could be put down to the loss of testosterone, rather than to the cancer. 'I used to lift four sheets of plasterboard no problem,' he told me, 'but I think I'll be lucky if I can manage two.' Over subsequent weeks his testicles shrank, and though he didn't lose the density of his beard his skin took on a pink, delicate sheen, as if it were becoming more fragile.

'Have you had enough?' I asked him one day, after he'd detailed all the side effects that were troubling him. 'Do you want to stop the treatment?'

'Not if it's doing me good,' he replied. 'If it's keeping down the cancer, for me at least – it's worth it.'

ALEX STILL ATTENDS my clinic every twelve weeks for the injections which wither his testicles but slow the growth of his tumour. A pragmatist by nature, he sees the exchange as a reasonable compromise: 'I'm lucky to be here,' he says, as he loosens his belt for the injections which, for their size, have to be given into the largest muscle in the body – the buttock.

After the initial shock of the treatment his libido returned, slowly, and one day he told me he had a new girlfriend. 'Her eyes are wide open,' he said, 'she knows I might not be around for ever.' I told him just to let me know if he wanted to try medication for impotence, but he just winked: 'no need,' he said, 'I've just got to use a bit more imagination than I used to.'

SOME MEN PERCEIVE the loss of testosterone as a punishing humiliation. Castration has long been exploited as punitive: the Oracle Bones of the Shang Dynasty in China, carved around 1500–1400 BCE, list castration as a sentence for prisoners of war, and an Egyptian Pharaoh who lived a couple of centuries later boasted of having castrated more than six thousand soldiers of an invading Libyan army. More recently, the Janjaweed militia in Sudan perpetrated the same on their prisoners. Some western jurisdictions today order chemical castration as a combined punishment and 'treatment' for convicted sex offenders, with controversial results.

Given the cultural hinterland of castration as punishment, it's a mystery as to why, historically, many young men and boys volunteered for such an ordeal. In *The Castrato*, a comprehensive examination of the phenomenon, the historian Martha Feldman explores some of the reasons why they did so. She proposes that we think of the exchange as much more than a bargain, but rather as a *sacrifice* – the transformation being in some sense sanctifying or sacralising. The castrato was offering something precious as a gift to celebrate the greater glory of God, but also in the hope of receiving something precious in return. Castrati, says Feldman, were 'sacralized creatures', in a way comparable to kings. In Confucian China that sacrifice was made to the state, and in Renaissance Italy, the church. It was seen as a kind of rebirth, much as Broyard felt that his life was given back to him when he received his terminal diagnosis.

Sir Thomas Browne noticed that after undergoing castration, males seemed to increase their chances of a long life – in part because diseases of the prostate had been neutralised. The Roman poet Lucretius, in *The Nature of Things*, describes sufferers of the plague sacrificing their testicles in the hope that they'd avoid the disease. Matthew's Gospel reads:

> There are some eunuchs, which were so born from their mother's womb: and there are some eunuchs, which were made eunuchs of men: and there be eunuchs, which have made themselves eunuchs for the kingdom of heaven's sake.

And there are some who choose castration in the hope of prolonging their lives.

20

Laughter: Some Eminency in Ourselves

We will try to avoid the error of those who in their subtle
disquisitions on the comic idea forgot that laughter is a bodily act.

James Sully, *An Essay on Laughter*, 1902

AT EIGHTEEN I HAD A JOB as a nursing assistant at a long-
stay residential hospital specialising in learning disabilities.
I wore a lemon-yellow uniform, and my job was to bathe
and dress male residents and help them with their meals.
The hospital had been built in the late 1960s, with four
hundred beds for the long-term care of those labelled
'mentally deficient'. Many had entered as children; I met
one who'd been committed for stealing a bicycle, another
told me he'd been locked up for climbing on roofs. Both,
as children, had been slow at school, and their parents had
complained of bad behaviour at home. My colleagues said
it was doubtful whether they'd manage now beyond the
walls of the hospital. I learned the bitter reality of the word
'institutionalised'.

For some of the residents there was a genetic background to their difficulties: it was my job to feed a boy with
Cornelia de Lange syndrome, who didn't have any hands
and couldn't speak. Every morning I'd help dress an elderly

man with Fragile X syndrome, a genetic disorder that may lead to learning disabilities. I struggled to get his legs into his trousers or socks on his feet – he had a beatific, amiable tolerance of my clumsiness. The other assistants knew that I was a medical student and at tea break they'd ask me about the details of genetic syndromes, or the drugs we helped dish out. I couldn't help them (I was in first year) but the job, and their enquiries, forced on me an early appreciation of the subtlety and fragility of the mind. Our brains are delicately calibrated, I realised, and there's a multiplicity of ways in which their potential can be frustrated. I had been living independently for only a few months; now I had an insight into the lives of those who never do.

On the ward was Henry, who according to the notes had the intellect and speech of a three-year-old. He had a bald head, stubby yellowed teeth, and a nose like a Roman general, as well as a tremendous and uninhibited capacity to laugh. He had a powerful, resplendent laugh, deep and sonorous, which he delivered sporadically throughout the day. When he wasn't laughing he'd usually be smiling – his expression at rest was one of irrepressible mirth. He loved dancing and music – the accordion music of Jimmy Shand was a favourite – and when music was playing he would take to the floor and whirl me around until he was gasping in great gales of laughter – I'd end up laughing alongside him. Afterwards, we'd sit back down to catch our breath, and there was a sense of some tension having been released, of some appreciable change for the better.

Now and again, in the throes of a full-bellied laugh, something would come over Henry, and that laughter would turn to a sob. Tears would bead at the corners of his eyes, and a choke would catch at his voice. 'What's the matter,' I'd ask him, 'is anything wrong?' He'd shake his head, shoulders shuddering, and I'd wait. A few moments later he'd be chuckling again, as if life was a joke to which tears or laughter were equally appropriate.

THERE ARE BROADLY TWO KINDS of laughter: the kind that floods out in response to something funny, and the kind of laugh that we put into conversation, to ease social interaction. As we get older we get better at distinguishing the two – the ability to tell the difference goes on improving into our forties. Both kinds of laughter are the ally of health: those who laugh regularly report less pain, anxiety and depression than others, as well as better sleep, energy and feelings of well-being. Laughter dilates blood vessels, dwindles heart disease and rallies our immune systems, making us less allergic but better able to fight infections. Many paediatric hospitals employ clowns, or 'giggle doctors', to ease tension and aid healing among attending children. 'Laughter is the best medicine,' goes the joke, 'unless you've got diarrhoea.'

We don't have much idea as to why we laugh. It's evidently a physical process – breathing is disturbed, the face becomes flushed, and we've all known the feeling of our sides aching with laughter. And there are mysterious physical changes associated with hearty laughter – I've known patients for whom a comedy show invariably brings on an asthma attack.

In 1900, the French philosopher Henri Bergson wrote an essay that was later translated as *Laughter: An Essay on the Meaning of the Comic*. For Bergson, human beings live in two worlds: the physical world that we perceive with the senses, and the social world of meanings, hierarchies, love, hate and mockery. He thought we laugh only in company, which isn't true – we do laugh alone, but we are thirty times more likely to laugh when we're with others, particularly with people we like, and who we want to like us (hence the 'canned' laughter on sitcom soundtracks). As human beings, he went on, we're on shifting social sands, constantly trying to figure out where we are situated with respect to those around us. Laughter reconciles us to the fact that we're changing social animals in a restless world;

it allows us to smooth the roughness of dynamic social exchange. It's cathartic of social tensions, and its work is to reinforce connections between individuals. Absent from Bergson's sophisticated theory is any robust attempt to integrate theories of laughter with the evident truth that small children laugh often, and with gusto, long before they've developed the intellect required to understand the meanings of jokes or care much about the opinions of others.

Charles Darwin, that master of unprejudiced observation, begins his study of 'high spirits' with children in mind: 'Laughter seems primarily to be the expression of mere joy or happiness. We clearly see this in children at play, who are almost incessantly laughing.' Laughter can also be provoked when there are incongruities between different associations of meaning, such as in the classic gag by Mae West: 'Marriage is a great institution, but I'm not ready for an institution.' Babies can be just as sensitive as adults to incongruities – a baby who laughs when she sees a tower of blocks fall over is observing that one moment the tower is stable, and the next it isn't – it could be the non-verbal discontinuity that provokes the laughter. Tickling too involves a kind of incongruity, as it's a mock 'attack' by a trusted person. Darwin thought a great deal about tickling:

> The anthropoid apes, as we have seen, likewise utter a reiterated sound, corresponding with our laughter, when they are tickled, especially under the armpits ... Yet laughter from a ludicrous idea, though involuntary, cannot be called a strictly reflex action. In this case, and in that of laughter from being tickled, the mind must be in a pleasurable condition; a young child, if tickled by a strange man, would scream from fear.

Darwin noticed that the movements involved in laughter – short, interrupted vocalisations on breathing out, with long drawn-out gasps on breathing in – are the precise opposite of those uttered when screaming with distress – so laughter acts as a powerful social signal of good humour. The transformative effect of a gale of laughter imposes a temporary paralysis that renders other actions, or the communication of other emotions, impossible.

Laughter to ease social relationships can be fake, or exaggerated, but it still serves a useful purpose. It marks our alignment or disalignment with others, and displays our affinity with those around us much more quickly than is possible with words. Aristotle thought that getting amused was a virtuous, social activity, as long as it was carried to the right extent, at the right time. He even had a word for it, *eutrapelia*, coming from the Greek meaning 'able to turn well'. If individuals can be imagined as cogs in a social machine, wittiness and humour are the grease that enables the machine to turn smoothly.

FOR HENRY, the frontier between tears of sorrow and tears of laughter was permeable and fragile – the two emotions seemed to have a common origin, and merge seamlessly from one to the other. One of oldest surviving books of medical case studies, the *Epidemics* of Hippocrates, noted how laughter and tears may erupt spontaneously in situations of extreme stress, almost as if they are interchangeable methods of coping: 'she used to wrap herself up … scratching and plucking out hair, and alternately wept and laughed.' Darwin commented that these transitions between tragedy and comedy, even in prominent social situations, are widespread among other cultures: 'Mr. Swinhoe informs me that he has often seen the Chinese, when suffering from deep grief, burst out into hysterical fits of laughter.' In western cultural traditions those rapid transitions between tears and laughter are restricted for the most part to babies and toddlers, though in situations of extreme stress they're observed in adults too. Darwin cites the 'recent' siege of Paris (his book was published in 1872): 'the German soldiers, after strong excitement from exposure to extreme danger, were particularly apt to burst out into loud laughter at the smallest joke.' Many people report the impulse to laugh at funerals, for example, not out of insensitivity, but from some inarticulate need for catharsis and to release tension from the grief of the situation. Perhaps the humour in bleak comedies arises from a similar kind of discomfort.

Among neurologists, the common origin of tears and of laughter is widely accepted – in the 1920s a syndrome called PLC, 'Pathological Laughter and Crying', was described: uncontrollable episodes of laughter or crying, or both at the same time, triggered by the most insignificant stimuli. For someone with PLC, sobs of distress might be provoked by having a hand waved in front of your eyes, or fits of giggles brought on by being given a plate of food. PLC can result from stroke, certain kinds of epilepsy, brain tumours, multiple sclerosis, and even the infusion of antiepileptic drugs, and seems quite separate from any subjective sense of mirth or well-being. It's apparently triggered by the activation of a kernel of tissue near the base of the brain that coordinates the muscular movements involved in both kinds of emotional expression. It's likely that the idiosyncrasies of Henry's brain led to the activation of this centre on the slightest of stimuli. The cerebellum – the 'little brain' beneath the nape of the neck – is also involved in laughter in some way: one of its functions is to coordinate not just appropriate movement, but the appropriateness of emotional expression.

In 1903, a French neurologist described a syndrome of *Fou rire prodromique* – 'anticipatory crazy laughter'. In this case uncontrollable, unemotional laughter caused by disinhibition of the brain centre was the herald to a stroke that led on rapidly to death. In an afterthought to his long poem Briggflatts, Basil Bunting relates a Persian tale of a stone in Tibet, the mere sight of which causes any viewer to descend into paroxysms of laughter 'which continues till they die'.

MANY YEARS AFTER I'd stopped working as a nursing auxiliary, I had a job providing medical cover to a hospice. Whenever I passed the day room there would be a funny movie, or a stand-up comedy routine, playing on the television. After the nurses took around their trolley of pills and suppositories, a trolley of comedy DVDs followed – a consolation, even a tonic, for patients and clinicians alike. Tea breaks and ward rounds were informal affairs – you could tell that the staff of the hospice were devoted to their work. There were just a few yards of hospital linoleum to walk between each bedside, but on passing between patients we would traverse mountain ranges of emotions. At one bedside there'd be solemnity, sadness and a frank discussion of death's approach; at the next we'd all be chuckling about constipation, or the eccentricities of hospital wheelchairs.

The philosopher Thomas Hobbes thought that laughter was a 'sudden glory arising from some sudden conception of some eminency in ourselves'. If he was right, perhaps there was laughter in the hospice to show superiority to the imminence of death. There was plenty of cathartic laughter to relieve tension; perhaps without it we could have been paralysed or overburdened by pity. We laughed at the absurdities and incongruities thrown up by the proximity of death in a society which reveres youth and health. We'd sometimes laugh to share solidarity with both colleagues and patients, and I'd sometimes hear laughter erupt from rooms at visiting time, perhaps easing tension between members of a family already wrapped in grief. The laughter wasn't cynical, or hard-hearted – it was changing the atmosphere, giving courage and a sense of togetherness, helping patients, doctors and relatives adapt to a new reality, when words no longer seemed enough.

21

Prosthetics: Humanity 2.0

He walked on an orthopaedic limb, but in such a manly way that
everyone envied him his walk.

Osip Mandelstam, Journey to Armenia

LIGHTSABERS MUST HAVE cauterising powers; when Luke
Skywalker lost a hand in *The Empire Strikes Back* the
stump hardly bled. Before long he had a new robotic hand,
whirring and clicking to that stump's commands. It's an old
idea that technology can restore us following mutilations,
and perhaps even give us an upgrade. Long John Silver and
Captain Ahab had their peg-legs, Captain Hook his eponymous hook. Pliny the Elder writes of a Roman general
during the Punic Wars who, following a traumatic amputation on the battlefield, had a prosthetic arm fashioned to
fit into his shield. One of the earliest literary forerunners
of Luke Skywalker's amputation is the moment in Ovid's
Metamorphoses when Pelops is hacked to pieces by his
father. The gods reconstitute his scattered parts, but can't
find the shoulder – they craft instead a replacement from an
elephant tusk 'making his body by such means complete'.

As a junior trainee in vascular surgery I used to assist
in limb amputations. Despite the sophistication of the hospital and the surgical implements it was always a surprise

how much of a grisly business it remained. As soon as the patient was anaesthetised, the cleavers and bone saws came out, and within minutes a severed limb would lie purpling on the green surgical drapes, before being tossed into an incinerator bag. The following morning, on the ward round, we'd check the stitching of the stumps, and make arrangements to introduce each patient to his or her prosthetist who'd fit them for a new limb. There was a new amputation every couple of weeks, usually performed because of blocked arteries – these were patients who'd suffered years of chronic pain and infections. On those crisp, starched, hospital sheets I'd see them gaze on their newly lightened, truncated limbs, stunned by the change effected on their bodies.

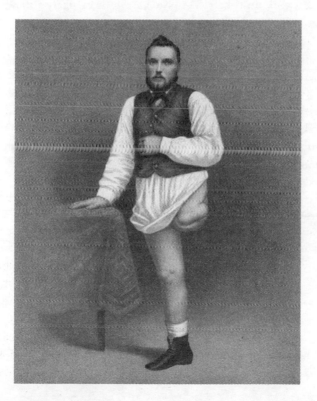

The earliest-known prosthesis is a big toe, made of wood and leather and found on the mummified foot of an Egyptian noblewoman buried three and a half thousand years ago. A bronze and iron leg dating from 300 BCE was unearthed two millennia later in southern Italy (it was transported to London, and destroyed during the Blitz). It's not until the early sixteenth century that there are stories of customised prosthetic hands – a German mercenary knight called Götz von Berlichingen lost his right arm in battle at the age of twenty-four, and had a replacement one built of iron, housing springs and pulleys. He went on to fight for Charles V against the Turks and the French. Armourers were the finest craftsmen of prostheses through the Middle Ages; they were the most skilled in ergonomic metalwork and their clients were the most likely to suffer amputations.

By the late sixteenth century, the Parisian surgeon Ambroise Paré was making sophisticated advances in prosthetic technology. He had noticed that people whose lives he saved through amputation often struggled with shame and disability, so he invented lifelike peg-legs that could kneel, and elbows that could bend. He also manufactured a hand with bendable fingers, and made prosthetic noses for those who had suffered nasal amputations.

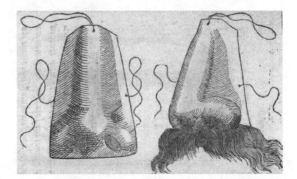

In one of the many conflicts between the Ottoman Empire and the Bulgarians, captured Ottoman soldiers had their noses amputated as a humiliation and a warning. It's said that on their return to Istanbul, the Sultan awarded each one an upgrade: a new nose cast in gold.

ANDREW GANNON HAS WORN a prosthetic arm for as long as he can remember – he was born with a left arm that ended at the elbow, and his parents insisted, even as a toddler, that he wear a prosthesis – keen that from his earliest years he'd build a mental self-image that included the limb he was born without. By age four, his prostheses were 'myoelectric'; that is, they could sense activity in the muscles of his arm and make the hand open or close accordingly.

On his left arm Andrew wears an 'iLimb', the latest of his myoelectric prostheses; it's sheathed in translucent silicon, revealing a skeletal intricacy of jointed and pistoned steel. The translucence of the prosthetic skin allows the branding over the back of the hand to be seen. It made a low electronic whine as Andrew demonstrated its capacities for me. 'There's so much pride in their engineering that the manufacturers want everyone to be able to see it,' he explained of the translucent glove, and shrugged; 'I'd rather just have it black.'* The silicon wears through quickly, exposing the robotics within to moisture, so he had to regularly change the cover. Some prosthetic limbs are now sheathed in photovoltaic cells, so that they can at least partially recharge as they are being used.

Andrew had had the iLimb for two years when we met. It has only two sensors within its socket – one over the muscles that would ordinarily work to open the hand, and one over the muscles that would ordinarily close the hand. The limb is plugged into an electric socket to charge every night. The vast range of potential movements programmed

---

* Since we met, Andrew has sourced a supply of plain black gloves.

into its circuits are initiated by just four signals: there's one signal to open the hand, initiated by a rapid muscular impulse at the elbow; a double impulse of the same signal; a triple impulse of open signal; and simultaneous contraction of both open and closing signal ('co-contraction'). The prosthesis switches between different programmes through sensing quickly alternating combinations of those signals: 'There was funding available to supply just two of these limbs in the region,' he told me. 'The prosthetic centre chose me because they knew I'd use it, and that I'd be honest in my feedback.' Initially he struggled with the complex movements required. 'But I got there in the end,' he said, reaching for a packet of paper tissues. Almost absent-mindedly, he held the crumpled plastic wrapping with the fingers of his iLimb, and pulled a tissue out with ease. 'That's one of the best things about this limb,' he said, noticing my gaze, 'the lateral grip. As a boy I had my own way of tying shoelaces, but this is the first limb that can manage the thumb movements involved in pulling out a tissue, or tightening a lace.'

The iLimb fingers have sensors within them that stop contracting when they meet resistance, meaning that Andrew can pick up an empty aluminium can without difficulties – previous limbs lacked sensitivity, and would crush cans in their grip. He uses both of his hands naturally in gestural body language, spreading wide open palms or closing his fist in context as he speaks. He also has an application on his smartphone that can wirelessly switch the limb between different settings, rendering the hand capable of positions such as the hold required to shake hands, or even make obscene gestures. But he rarely uses these – the four pre-set programmes are enough. 'I've a new baby at home,' he told me, 'but I decided against changing nappies with the limb. It's quicker and safer just to slip the limb off, finish the nappy one-handed, and then put the limb back on.'

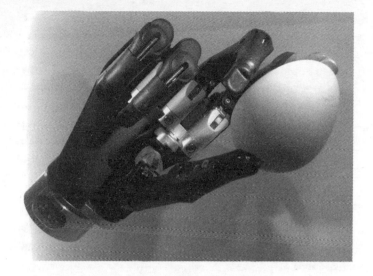

THERE ARE AN ESTIMATED four million people around the world who have suffered amputation of a limb – only a tiny proportion of them are rich enough (or live in countries rich enough) to afford myoelectric prostheses. Olivia Giles is a quadruple amputee living in Edinburgh; in 2002 she lost her hands and feet to a rare form of meningitis which causes blood poisoning. Trained as a lawyer, she now works full time as the director of the charity 500 Miles, providing prosthetic limbs in Malawi and Zambia.

I asked about her own experience, losing her hands and feet to septicaemia a decade earlier. A bacterial infection in the bloodstream had reduced the circulation to her extremities so profoundly that they had turned gangrenous, and had to be amputated. 'One day at work I felt really ill, as if I had flu,' she said. 'The following morning I saw these purple spots spreading over my feet, and then my hands, and felt dreadful – I went to the hospital where I collapsed unconscious. Then I woke up four weeks later like this' – she raised her forearms that end short of the wrists. 'I came within an inch of dying, but I survived, and that's why I've never looked back. I've more regrets about my life before the amputations than I do about the life I've lived since.'

I asked Olivia about the transition to her new life – for many people who suffer amputations, the first few months or even years can be torturous. 'The day I got up on my prosthetic legs and took a couple of steps was like a rebirth – the beginning of a new life,' she said. 'I was euphoric; I hadn't dared to hope that one day I might walk out of hospital. So almost immediately I began thinking about a charity, so that others could have the same chance for a second life as I've had. Malawi is a place with great need, and it isn't war-torn – when I chose a place to start the charity I wanted to be able to visit and supervise it myself. And Zambia – there are so many strong connections between Scotland, Malawi and Zambia.'

I was surprised that the majority of the charity's work was to offer prosthetic legs; arms were lower priority. 'For an adult, in sub-Saharan Africa, they know they will never be given a job over someone who is able-bodied,' Olivia said. 'Once they've had an amputation their life as a working adult is largely over, but prostheses can enable them to go on working in the fields. We fit arm prostheses that have sprung hooks that can hold a hoe or a rake, but legs give people mobility, which means freedom. The arms that we use are really just cosmetic – people get mocked and ostracised, and supplying a dummy limb can help them to fit in.' Olivia told me that someone who has lost one arm still has around 95 per cent of their ability to function – adding a prosthetic arm, even a sophisticated one like an iLimb, adds only an extra 5 per cent.

'The most transformative thing about prosthetic limbs is the potential they offer for children,' she told me. 'The kids we work with, if they lose a limb in an accident, they become trapped in the home, a burden on their families, often ashamed of the disfigurement. Having a prosthetic leg makes it possible for them to go back to school. You can see it in the mothers' faces when the new limbs are fitted, their faces light up, because they know that this means that their child has a future. The prosthesis gives them a future.'

The limbs that Olivia's charity supplies are made in Switzerland, not locally in Africa; she told me that the locally sourced limbs are not yet of high-enough quality. 'We order them in batches, then ship them out to Lusaka and Blantyre and Lilongwe,' she said. The local prosthetists she employs have all studied on a diploma course in Cambodia; as a consequence of the war there, low-cost prosthetic technology is advanced. 'It'd be cheaper to have the prosthetists train over in Tanzania,' she added, 'but the course isn't yet as good. There's a diploma course too in Togo, but it's French-speaking, which is no good for our Zambians and Malawians.'

Over the years, I've known many amputees struggle with phantom pain, prejudiced attitudes about disability, chronic depression and anxiety. But Olivia was upbeat about the possibilities open to amputees, even those who have suffered multiple amputations like herself: 'We're so lucky to live in a western society where it's acceptable to be disabled, where society has made accommodations for us, where there's legislation, where things are accessible. It's possible to have a high quality of life here in Scotland no matter your disability. The facilities and the funds available in the UK are generous: here, if the mould for your stump doesn't quite fit then it's discarded and a new one is made. That would never happen in poorer countries where they have to make do with what they've got.'

The charity doesn't only provide prosthetic limbs, it issues splints to straighten club feet, and orthotics to help burned skin heal without disfiguring and disabling contractures. 'Some don't realise how important it is to look after the skin of a burn,' she said. 'Many hospitals in Africa have a terrible reputation, and people tend to run away as soon as they can. We're working hard to convince people of the importance of good follow-up.'

Olivia is positive about the possibilities of life after amputation; that even simple, low-cost prosthetics can revolutionise lives for the better. 'It doesn't make any sense to me how someone could look at me and my body, and feel pity, when my body is healthy and strong! How much more miserable would it be to have chronic depression, or a degenerative condition that you can't see but which is going to shorten your life. My life isn't going to be shorter because of having no hands and no feet – it's just a little more inconvenient.'

WITH TECHNOLOGY, humanity has the opportunity not just to replace the function of a missing limb, but to improve on it. The word *prosthesis* means 'addition' – hidden in the word's root is the hint that prostheses might enhance the possibilities of human beings, rather than just substituting them. Pelops had a replacement shoulder carved from ivory; now prosthetists use titanium, carbon fibre, and Kevlar.

Many years ago I met Jamie Andrew, a quadruple amputee who lost both hands and both feet to frostbite in an Alpine climbing accident. Like Olivia, he prefers not to use prosthetic hands from day to day. 'I think you've got to ask yourself what the limb is for,' he told me. 'Is it to replace a missing part – because you're never going to get back your hand – or is it a tool to help you do things?' Jamie leaned forwards, deftly picked up his coffee cup with his handless forearms, and took a sip. 'If it's a tool, well, I have plenty of those, and they work better than hands. I have an arm designed for driving, arms for ice climbing, an arm with a kitchen knife for chopping vegetables … I could go on. All these are better at their function than my hands were.'

'And the new generation of myoelectric limbs?' I asked

him. 'What do you think about the value, the usefulness of those?'

'I'd be more interested in the technology if they tried to make an improvement on the human hand, instead of trying to make a slower, clunkier, second-class copy of one.'

A few years ago one of the UK's military prosthetic centres closed, and its funding was passed over for use through the UK National Health Service. The transfer meant that civilians had access to the kind of technology that previously was available only to veterans. 'Take rock climbing, for example,' said Jamie. 'My climbing legs have stubby little toe-fronts on their feet that are perfect for narrow crevices in the rock. Or skiing: human thighs, knees and calves are pretty good at absorbing pressure from uneven snow surfaces. My old skiing legs had sprung carbon-fibre dampeners, which worked well, but would chatter over the ice on sharp turns. But my latest skiing legs have mini shock absorbers, like the ones that you see on the front forks of a bicycle – they're perfect for eliminating vibration, and better than a human leg.'

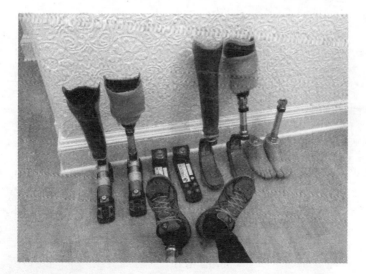

I told Jamie that I'd heard there was disagreement in the amputee community about the value of pursuing transplants, versus the value of concentrating on developing and refining prostheses. The reality of 3D scanning of stumps, and 3D printing to build sockets, allied to an ever-evolving toolkit of synthetic materials, means that Paralympic athletes are catching up with able-bodied ones – in some instances they surpass them. It's as if prosthetics might offer more than just a replacement for a missing limb, but a new improved version of being human – Humanity 2.0. Jamie laughed: 'If someone was to offer me a hand like Luke Skywalker's I'd take it,' he said, 'though that's a long way off.' But not light years away.

22

Memory: Palaces of Forgetting

One condition of remembering is that we should forget.

William James, *The Principles of Psychology*

THE FOURTH CALL of the night shift was to a nursing-home resident, George B., who the staff said had become uncharacteristically belligerent. Earlier in the day he'd struck out at another resident of the home – something he'd never done before. It was turning into a busy night: the first call had been to give morphine to a woman on her deathbed. She had looked as if she might not survive until morning, and the morphine had helped ease her pain and breathlessness. The second was to decide if a man had dislocated his artificial hip, but he met me at the door with little more than a limp. The third was to a young woman who'd phoned the service in a panic, hallucinating that her living-room carpet was infested with spiders. It turned out that she wasn't psychotic – she had just been injecting amphetamines.

I pushed a buzzer and stood at the door next to a rusting municipal bench and a bin for stubbing out cigarettes. It was a modern construction in cheap brown brick, all on one level, with a peaked gable roof over the entrance. On the glass door there were notices asking me not to disturb residents at mealtimes, to sign in and out of the building, and please remember to sterilise my hands. I peered in through the glass: a mandatory fish tank, scrubbable carpets, wipeable easy chairs, and information boards with photographs of the staff, alongside montage illustrations of residents on days away. As I waited, an angular, elderly woman in a dressing gown appeared on the other side of the glass. She was leaning with determination over a walking frame, and stopped for a moment to look through at me. Her left hand went up in a regal salute, then she smiled a dazzling, hundred-watt smile. For a second or two we stood smiling at one another. Then she moved on down the corridor, looking from side to side as she went, like a queen surveying the splendour of her palace.

It was another couple of minutes before a nurse flustered to the door to let me in. Her hair was in a high bun with a pen stabbed through it, and her dark-blue uniform told me that she was in charge for the night. In one hand she held a bunch of keys, and in the other a sheaf of papers in plastic wallets. 'I'm Maggie – sorry for the wait,' she said, turning on her heels and striding back in the direction she'd come from. She gestured for me to follow: 'short-staffed,' she added.

'Don't worry,' I said.

I caught up with her at another set of double doors. 'George is usually so mild-mannered' – she punched a code into a keypad on the wall – 'a real gentleman.' We were stopped as the door opened: a frail, bowed man wearing a green polo shirt and nothing below the waist met us at the door. 'I'm just going home,' he said, 'see you,' and pushed past me into the main corridor.

'Not that way, Jimmy,' said Maggie, lunging to catch him. She took him persuasively by the arm, directing without forcing him down a separate corridor – he clearly trusted her. 'Go and get your trousers, please,' she said to him, then grinned at me. 'Welcome to the madhouse,' she said in a stage whisper.

In this half of the building there were only men – several were walking up and down the corridor, some were sitting in a lounge. They all looked clean and well cared for. On an unwatched television, celebrities walked down a red carpet; the room flickered with the flashbulbs of paparazzi.

Maggie led me down the corridor to George's room. 'Carol will look after you,' she said, and strode off again at a clipped pace. George's name and his photograph were tacked to the door: a big man, bald, with a summer shirt open to the waist, bronzed and smiling into the camera. A holiday snapshot. His shoulders were muscled, and his tattooed arms were stretched around a wife, daughters, grandchildren.

The room inside had been stripped of anything that could be used as a weapon, and in its centre George lay naked on a bed. He was paler and more haggard than his photograph. Arrayed around the walls were photocopies of old photographs. George in uniform, medals on his broad chest; one standing by a jeep, another of him saluting a senior officer. There was a close-up photograph of the same medals taken decades later, I presumed: they were tarnished and dusty. George lay on his back, eyes open, fingertips held to his cheeks. Sweat beaded on his forehead and his lips moved as if in silent prayer. There was no sign of Carol.

I put my bag down next to the bed. 'Hello, George,' I said, 'I'm Gavin Francis, the doctor. How are you?' I took his right hand off his cheek gently, as if to shake it, and with my left felt for his pulse. A middle-aged woman in the yellow tunic of a nursing assistant stepped out of the adjoining bathroom. She had white bobbed hair and drawn-on eyebrows. 'He won't reply,' she said, 'he's hardly spoken all day.' She moved to the other side of his bed and put a hand on his shoulder. 'You're not right, are you, George? Poor love.' Her voice was sing-song, as if speaking to a child, but the affection in it was honest. We both stood for a moment looking down on his naked body in all its tragic strength, so deserted by his mind. I looked away, up at the photographs on the walls, and Carol followed my gaze. 'He was a captain in the army,' she said. 'He told me that one' – she pointed up at the photograph of George saluting the more senior officer – 'was taken in Berlin, just after the war ended. He can still tell you all about his medals.'

I nodded. 'Haven't you got a sheet for him?'

'He just throws them off,' Carol said. She pointed at some clothing in the corner; 'His pyjamas need a wash.'

I leaned in closer to George's ear: 'I'm just going to check your temperature and examine you,' I said. He showed no sign of having heard, and his lips muttered on. I pushed the nozzle of a thermometer into his ear, and its reading showed a slight fever. Bending over him, I put my stethoscope to his chest: the air moved cleanly through his lungs, his heart murmured as if an unoiled cog was turning slowly inside. I took off the stethoscope and began gently to press on his belly, and he winced. 'Did you manage to get a urine sample?' I asked Carol.

'In there,' she said, pointing her thumb over her shoulder into the bathroom. I took the urine testing sticks from my bag and went in: tough-wearing institutional lino; a hard plastic chair beneath a disability shower; handles on the walls; polythene-wrapped packets of incontinence pads.

To assess whether urine has an infection takes a full two minutes – those one hundred and twenty seconds can be the only slack moments in a shift. Urine testing sticks have tiny squares of chemical reagents on them; after those chemicals are dipped in urine they change colour, coming to resemble the swatches of paint in a DIY store, or the colour-keys to altitude in the corner of old maps. Sometimes, as I wait, I'm conscious of the centuries of physicians before me who have scrutinised urine for clues. Usually I just watch the colours evolve. Sometimes I remember the clinical exam, many years ago now, when a distinguished professor asked me to dip a urine stick and hold it out, 'so I can see if your hands are shaking'.

I dipped the thin paper testing stick into the urine Carol had left out on the sink and, glancing at my watch, counted out thirty seconds before the urine's sugar level could be gauged, a minute to read off its blood and protein, two minutes to assess its white blood cells. The protein square turned the pale green of the nursing-home corridors. The white blood cell square turned the same lilac as the shower curtain.

The combination of lilac, green and some streaks of midnight blue confirmed that George had another urine infection. The workings of his brain were so tenuously balanced that just a few bacteria growing in his bladder, and the associated toxins in his blood, had tipped this ordinarily gracious if forgetful man into terror and bewilderment.

No one understands the exact mechanism which makes people with dementia so vulnerable to a worsening of memory when they have an infection. In medical terminology George had a 'delirium', a particular species of confusion named for a Latin word referring to ploughing: 'delirare' means 'out of furrow'. George's brain and mind were accustomed to well-worn routines and habitual responses; the urine infection had jolted the ploughshare of his mind from its customary track.

IN 1943 THE THEORETICAL PHYSICIST Erwin Schrödinger gave a series of lectures at Trinity College Dublin entitled 'What is Life?' He dedicated the lectures, and the book that came of them, to the memory of his parents. For Schrödinger, our ability to learn and hold memories was what most made us human. The brain and central nervous system, he explained, were engaged in the constant 'phylogenetic transformation' of learning. To learn something new was to be engaged in a deep and intimate way with your own humanity.

Schrödinger delivered another series of lectures thirteen

years later, at Trinity College Cambridge. He titled them *Mind and Matter*, and elaborated on his Dublin theme: much of what we consider the self is intimately connected to our ability to make new memories, which we use to build images of both present and future. Loss of memory may lead to a loss of self; memory is how we weave the world into existence. 'There really is no before and after for mind,' he wrote. 'There is only a now that includes memories and expectations.'

Schrödinger was schooled in the classics and begins a memorable passage in *Mind and Matter* by comparing the neuroscience of consciousness with a scene in Homer's *Odyssey*, when a blind bard sings of the horrors of the war so beautifully that Odysseus begins to weep. The bard's name is Demodocus, which means 'honoured-by-the-people'; it's thought that Homer intended him as a self-portrait. Just as Homer's poem was a tapestry of epic magnificence with a self-portrait stitched into it, so Schrödinger said that our mind weaves experience from skeins of memories, then contrives to knit our conscious selves in as participants.

After reading Schrödinger's *Mind and Matter* I went to dig out the passage: 'It's as if you were present yourself at Troy, or have heard the tale from a witness,' says Odysseus to Demodocus. 'You must have been taught by the Muses or by Apollo.'

The 'Muses' were the daughters of Zeus and of Memory; the earliest sources have it that there were three of them: 'Meditation', 'Remembrance' and 'Song'.* The 'Museum' was their palace, and their work was to give inspiration, by infusing memories with a divine spark of creative life.

---

* Later sources speak of nine Muses, with fabulous names, including 'lovely-voice', 'make-famous', 'heavenly-one', 'give-delight', 'beloved', 'song-celebration', 'many-hymns', 'dance-delighting' and 'flourishing'.

MEMORY ALLOWS US to travel in time and space, it moors us in the present, liberates us from the moment, and offers to take us into the past, as well as imagine the future. Conversely, the loss of memory is socially isolating and profoundly disorientating; to lose memory is to experience a change in the nature of the self. There are a hundred billion cells in the human brain with an average of five thousand synapses each: five hundred trillion potential connections in which to embed memories. The scale and splendour of these neural networks took a long time to elucidate – neuronal branches ('dendrites') were too densely packed for the first microscopists to trace the connections of a single cell. It was like trying to visualise a single tree, wrapped in a thicket of thorns, in a rainforest, at night. In the late nineteenth century, a technique was developed by an Italian, Camillo Golgi, then improved by a Spaniard, Santiago Ramón y Cajal, that was capable of staining just a few neurons in a thin slice of brain tissue. It was as if a way had been found to select a few trees in that dark rainforest and charm them into luminescence. In drawings of magnificent elegance, Ramón y Cajal revealed the awesome complexity of the brain's networks of memory.

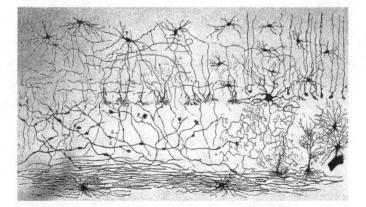

Neuroscientists speak of several ways in which we learn new memories. Impressions pass in milliseconds from our senses into the brain, and are then filtered through grids of semantic memory that make 'sense' of them – it's through the organising sieves of semantic memory, learned by experience over years, that sound becomes understood words, and patterns of light become recognisable images. Our brains do not passively sense the world – they knit it from moment to moment by braiding and knotting remembered encounters from the past. Those networks are continually modified as certain connections or 'synapses' are strengthened while others are weakened – a process called 'synaptic plasticity'. Plasticity entails material change to the structures around the synapse. Memories are sustained in part through a long-term modification of calcium and sodium channels in the membrane of each brain cell.

There are several distinct types of memory. It appears there's a dedicated network just for 'working memory'; reverberating loops of neural activity in the cortex which can hold information for just a few minutes. Nobody understands the fragile mechanism of this, or why it's so easily sidetracked. If you see a car perform a hit-and-run, you can be distracted from committing the car's colour and registration number to memory, but you can't be distracted from remembering the colour or registration of your own car.

The memory of what you were doing at the time of major events, such as 9/11, or the assassination of JFK, is termed a 'flashbulb memory'. Particular events of your remembered past are termed by neuropsychologists 'episodic memories': decisive, photographic moments in the narratives of our lives. Though these episodes too are little understood, it's known that the hippocampus – a baroque curl of cortex in the base of each temporal lobe – is fundamental to establishing them, and sleep is necessary to consolidate them. The hippocampus needs a lot of oxygen, which suggests that it's extraordinarily active; children who've suffered periods of oxygen starvation have fewer hippocampal neurons, and poorer memories as a consequence. One of neuropsychology's most famous patients, Henry Molaison ('H. M.'), had surgery to both hippocampi to mitigate epilepsy in 1953. He woke with fewer seizures but unable to commit any new experience to memory.

Other parts of the brain than the higher cortex and hippocampus are involved in alternative modes of memory. The basal ganglia that lie just beneath the cerebral hemispheres learn how to transform new deliberative movements and behaviours into seamless, unconscious actions. Timing of movements is 'remembered' elsewhere, in networks of the brain's cerebellum, which coordinates complex actions like speech, or delivering a serve at tennis. People with damage to the cerebellum have impaired working memories, suggesting that it is essential for coordinating words and images, not just muscles. The cells that accomplish this are among the most intricately branched neurons in the brain.

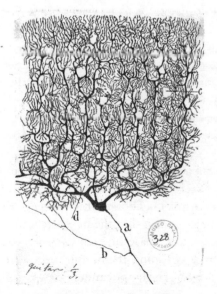

The forgetting of Henry Molaison was of a sudden and catastrophic kind – from the day of his surgery he was unable to remember anything new. The only comparable pathology in normal clinical practice is Korsakoff's psychosis – something I've seen only once in twenty years of practice – when a destructive alcoholism, in alliance with certain vitamin deficiencies, brings on irreversible brain damage. This is the kind of memory loss that afflicted 'Jimmie G.' in Oliver Sacks's essay 'The Lost Mariner' – a man cursed by Korsakoff's to be marooned in time while life flowed on around him. Jimmie G. was admitted to Sacks's hospital with a note saying only 'helpless, demented, confused and disorientated'. But Sacks found his personality intact, and his mind robust for everything but the creation of new memories.

To get a glimpse of the myriad ways of forgetting, it's worth glancing at the index of a textbook of psychiatry. Under dementia you might find 'alcoholic', 'Alzheimer's', 'cerebrovascular', 'Creuzfeldt-Jakob', 'depressive', 'Lewy Body', 'Parkinsonian', and 'psychotic'. Up to half of the dementia I see is 'cerebrovascular': as the body ages its blood vessels silt up and the result is a slower, more forgetful brain. Some is 'Parkinsonian': Parkinson's disease may progress from a difficulty initiating movements to a difficulty initiating thoughts and, eventually, memories. But in many who attend my clinic complaining of memory loss, a cause can't be identified – psychiatrists classify these as 'Alzheimer's type'. When post-mortem examinations are performed on the brains of people with this kind of dementia, memory circuits are seen to be clogged with two unusual proteins. The first, 'beta-amyloid', is found in plaques between the brain cells; the second, called 'tau', is found in tangles within the cells themselves.

The reason why these substances accumulate remains a mystery, and we know little about how to prevent them. The onset of forgetting in Alzheimer's is insidious: for many, the process moves so slowly that it never causes difficulties, while for others the accretion of tau and amyloid is accelerated for reasons that remain obscure. There are some drugs which, if started early, may slow the decline by about six months at best, but these too have side effects, and are often poorly tolerated by the frail, elderly people who need them most.

When Sacks sought the advice of the great Russian neuropsychologist A. R. Luria about how he might treat Jimmie G., he received an eloquent and compassionate response.

> There are no prescriptions in a case like this. Do whatever your ingenuity and your heart suggest. There is little or no hope of any recovery in his memory. But a man does not consist of memory alone. He has feeling, will, sensibilities, moral being – matters of which neuropsychology cannot speak. And it is here, beyond the realm of an impersonal psychology, that you may find ways to touch him, and change him. And the circumstances of your work especially allow this, for you work in a Home, which is like a little world, quite different from the clinics and institutions where I work. Neuropsychologically, there is little or nothing you can do; but in the realm of the Individual, there may be much you can do.

Luria's advice reads as a plea for dedicated, resource-rich nursing care for people with dementia; care that's possible in homes like the one I was called into in order to see George. In the absence of any effective treatment for memory loss, it's the quiet humanity and enthusiasm of nursing staff like Maggie and Carol that we have to support.

WE LIVE LONGER now than at any other time in the history of humanity, and dementia may seem like a modern epidemic. But it's nothing new. 'Nothing whatever, in man, is of so frail a nature as the memory', says Pliny's *Natural History* (c. 70 CE) 'for it is affected by disease, by injuries, and even by fright ... very often the memory appears to attempt, as it were, to make its escape from us, even while the body is at rest and in perfect health.' But dementia is of less interest to Pliny than its converse, the stories he'd heard of prodigious memories. He recounts the rumours about King Cyrus of the Persians, who was said to remember the names of every one of his thousands of soldiers; of an ambassador who within a day of arriving in Rome had memorised the names of every senator; and of a man called Charmidas, who, on being given the name of any book in the library, could recount it just as if he was reading aloud.

Jorge Luis Borges borrowed from Pliny for his story *Funes the Memorious*, in which a Uruguayan gaucho, Ireneo Funes, falls from a horse and wakes up crippled in body, but with a newly infallible memory. Through the power of perfect memory Funes' world is transformed to one of almost unbearable richness and brightness; the depths of his vaguest recollections become illuminated with brilliance and clarity. He becomes able to remember every configuration of clouds he has ever seen, and forms comparisons in his mind's eye between those skyscapes and all the varieties of marbled patterns he has ever glimpsed in the binding of books. In the back bedroom of his mother's house, working only by candlelight, Funes learns English, French, Portuguese and Latin simply by flicking through dictionaries. Borges has Funes declaiming Pliny in a flawless Latin learned only hours before.*

Normal life is impossible for Funes, distracted as he is by the variety and ceaseless metamorphosis of the

---

* There's a suggestion that Borges himself possessed a prodigious eidetic memory. Many years after he had become blind, he was able to remember the book, page and which part of the page, he had first seen a particular quotation.

world around him. The vivacity and lucidity of his visual memory means that he is tortured by the subtle effects of ageing, of entropy, of rot, of the creep that all living things make moment to moment into senescence. Memory is intimately bound to our humanity, but it has to be selective; an overactive and vivid memory can be a curse, and not just for savants like Funes. I've known many hundreds of patients unmoored by memory loss, but I've known dozens who would welcome the forgetting of painful memories. Forgetting can be just as important as remembering. 'The truth is,' concludes Borges's narrator, 'we all live by leaving behind.'

ON A HILL overlooking the nursing home where Maggie and Carol work there's a palatial university business school, set back from the road by a croquet lawn, and in it a small museum. It's not immediately obvious from the road, being hidden behind mature stands of chestnut, sycamore and Scotch pine. When I last visited it was spring: cherry blossom was out along the main road, and the croquet lawn was edged with bluebells. You wouldn't think you were in the midst of a city, and when the building was first constructed, it wasn't. It was designed in the style of an Italian palace as a 'hydropathic hospital' in the closing decades of the Victorian era, for fee-paying customers attracted by its peaceful location and a spring famous for its curative waters. The central tower has five storeys, the wings of it just three; high sash windows look north-west in the direction of Fife. In 1916 the hospital was requisitioned for the war effort and rechristened Craiglockhart War Hospital. Shell-shocked officers were sent there to recuperate following the atrocities of the Somme.

The small museum preserves the memory of how the building, between 1916 and 1919, was home to nearly two thousand officers – among them the poets Wilfred Owen and Siegfried Sassoon. One of the psychiatrists in residence,

William H. R. Rivers, pioneered a new approach to those tortured by their memories. Rather than accuse the officers of cowardice or malingering, Rivers sought to understand how these men's memories had become a torment, and how they might be induced to remember without pain.

In December 1917, Rivers addressed the Royal Society of Medicine in London on his work at Craiglockhart. To repress memories wasn't pathological, he said, but a 'necessary element in education and in all social progress'. Soldiers, said Rivers, usually learn over long periods of training to dampen their distress at war, and divert the powerful emotions generated in conflict into other channels. But the war had come too precipitously, and the training of the men had been inadequate: 'Training in repression normally spread over years has had to be carried out in short spaces of time,' Rivers wrote, 'while those thus incompletely trained have had to face strains such as have never previously been known in the history of mankind.' The problem in shell-shock was not repression *per se*, but maladaptive and ineffective repression. The only antidote to the poison of recurrent, traumatic memories was to bring them back into the light of remembrance, re-examine them with a psychiatrist, and hope that their emotional significance would fade.

One of Rivers' cases was an officer who had walked out into no man's land only to stumble over his friend's head, torso and limbs, ripped apart by a shell. The officer tried to forget the appalling incident, but every night as he slept was gripped by nightmares of seeing again his mutilated friend blasted across the battlefield. He'd wake in terror, sweat soaking his pillow. Rivers realised that it was the man's love for his friend which gave this horrific memory its power, and searched for some element of the experience that 'would allow the patient to dwell on it in such a way as to relieve its horrible and terrifying character'. He focused the man's reflections on the 'conclusive evidence that [his friend] had been killed outright, and had been spared the prolonged suffering which is too often the fate of those who suffer mortal wounds'.

According to Rivers, the man's face brightened at once: 'He saw that this was an aspect of his experience upon which he could allow his thoughts to dwell.' From that day, whenever the painful memory came to mind, he'd imbue it with the reassuring thought that his friend had been spared suffering. After a few nights the dream disappeared. Then it began again, but this time without fear or horror. In the second version of the dream he was able to direct his actions: he crouched down next to the dead friend, touched his belongings and gathered them, and was even able to converse gently with him about their shared grief.

In 1917, the year after Siegfried Sassoon was discharged from Craiglockhart, he contributed two poems to an anthology of war poetry, its title invoking those gods of Memory: *The Muse in Arms*. Throughout the anthology, there are images of war as a kind of delirium or madness. One of the poems contributed by Sassoon, 'The Rear-Guard', hints at a modest liberation achieved by leaving painful memories behind, though that liberation might be into death on the open battlefield:

> At last, with sweat and horror in his hair,
> He climbed through darkness to the twilight air,
> Unloading hell behind him, step by step.

AFTER CHECKING GEORGE'S URINE in the en-suite bathroom I moved back to his bedside. Carol was sitting beside him now, stroking his arm and talking in a low, soothing voice. 'He has a urine infection,' I said. 'I'll just go out to the car and get some antibiotics for him.' Before leaving, I stood watching George for a moment. He still showed no sign of having noticed me, his lips continued to murmur, and sweat pooled at the corners of his eyes. I wondered how much of his memory had been lost in tangles of beta-amyloid and tau proteins, yet Carol had told me that, when well, he was able to remember much about the war seventy years earlier, and the stories behind each of his medals. With luck the antibiotics would nudge him out of his delirium, back to the habitual furrows along which his thoughts and his memories ran. In a delirium of memory loss we can lose much of what we think of as identity; with treatment of his infection, and good care from staff like Carol, I hoped that George would find himself again.

Maggie led me back through three sets of doors, a different code punched in each time. We stepped out into the night. For a moment we stood together, savouring the moment of being between tasks, breathing open air. I walked over to the car, saw that two more visits had come through to the emergency services laptop, and picked up a box of antibiotics. On my way back towards the double doors I saw Maggie talking with the elderly lady I'd seen earlier – the one who had saluted me like a queen. She was explaining some urgent matter, eyes bright, hands animated. Maggie stood listening patiently, a hand on her shoulder, as if she had all night.

23

Death: The Celebration of Life

You can frighten people with death or an idea of their own mortality, or it can actually give them vigour.

Damien Hirst

A DETECTIVE INSPECTOR once told me that the key thing to remember at a crime scene was to keep your hands in your pockets; the temptation to reach out and touch a murder victim, or a potential murder weapon, could be overwhelming. He had little faith in forensic pathologists. 'I was at a scene where a dead man lay slumped over a desk,' he told me. 'There was a narrow entry wound on the back of his head, and a hole in the victim's forehead. A Bakelite phone on the desk was shattered into pieces – he had obviously been shot. The pathologist arrived: "Hmm," he said. "Looks like we're searching for a stiletto, or maybe a knife."'

Once he was called to a high-rise block of flats. A body had been found in an advanced state of decomposition. 'It was the strangest thing I've ever seen,' he told me. 'I had a witness saying she was alive only the day before, but the witness must have been wrong. There she was, turning into liquid.'

He had retired early, and I asked whether having dealt

with so many murders had made him pessimistic about life. 'Not pessimistic,' he said, 'but more philosophical. Enjoy it while it lasts.'

AFTER OUR BRIEF ENCOUNTERS in the clinic, my patients go out into the world, and it may be months or years until I see them again. Occasionally, I hear later from the hospital or the police that they've died. That death is usually in some way expected, or could at least have been anticipated. When death comes as a surprise, or is in some way suspicious, the body of the deceased goes for an autopsy, or post-mortem.

Recently, on the phone with a pathologist about a post-mortem report that she had prepared on one of my patients, I realised how rarely I had cause to speak to her or her colleagues. 'So much of my practice is guesswork,' I said to her, 'trying to figure out what's going on beneath my patients' skin. I envy you being able to take a look inside and figure out what's happening once and for all.' 'That's a misconception,' the pathologist, Charlotte Crichton, replied. 'We don't have all the answers either.' She invited me to come and see for myself.

I met Charlotte at 8.30 a.m. sharp, in her office, where she was busy with the police summaries for the morning's cases. There was a man whose body had been pulled from a river; fishing tackle had been found nearby. 'He might well have stumbled and drowned,' Charlotte said. There was a woman in her fifties, found dead on her sofa; Charlotte wanted to find out whether the woman had died of a heart attack, which seemed likely, or had been poisoned by gas or drugs. 'It's relatively unusual for us to do a post-mortem on a woman,' she said; 'it tends to be men who die violent or suspicious deaths.' Finally, there was a man with morbid obesity, found face down in his kitchen, who could conceivably have choked on some food he was preparing. The circumstances of each were detailed in a police report, listing witness statements, some medical history provided by the GP, and also any pertinent information provided by family members. There was a brisk professionalism about Charlotte's description of each patient, as well as an unmistakable curiosity. She was in the business of looking for answers, and hoped that the morning's work would deliver them.

I changed into blue hospital scrubs. Between the locker room and the autopsy suite was a tiled tray of the kind used to disinfect your feet at a swimming pool; rubber boots were lined up against the wall, next to a hose for washing them down. The suite was somewhere at the heart of the building and saw little natural light. There were three body-sized steel trays at waist height; when there were enough pathologists around, autopsies could be carried out three at a time. The ventilators in the ceiling were designed to push air down and away from the noses of the pathologists. 'At least that's the idea,' Charlotte said. 'It doesn't seem to work very well.' Along one side of the room was a glass wall with seating behind it: a viewing gallery for students. A fluorescent purple Insect-O-Cutor blinked high on one wall next to a sign: 'No eating, drinking or smoking.' We tied on disposable aprons, rolled plastic gauntlets up our sleeves, tucked the gauntlets into surgical gloves, and were ready to start.

The first time I ever saw a dead body was in the first week of medical school, in the dissection room. It was the body of a man, partly skinned. Most of him was obscured under a linen cloth, but his right arm, stiff with rigor mortis, pointed at the ceiling. Preservatives had turned the muscles brown; they spiralled from the hand towards the elbow like ivy around a tree trunk.

In the mortuary, the first dead body – let's call him Philip – was pulled out on a gurney. No linen cloth had been draped over him, no preservatives had been injected: his skin was grey and mottled, and for the most part intact, except where fish had nibbled. His eyes were half-open, and his head thrown back. The first task of the post-mortem examination was an external search for scratches, scars and injuries. Charlotte carefully examined his hands, nails and feet for evidence of a struggle, and pointed out that his right eye was bloodshot. 'But look: his arm is reddened on the right too. So it's only bloodshot from gravity, because he's been lying on that side after he died.'

Charlotte took a scalpel and made a long cut from the notch at Philip's throat to his pubic bone, and opened his abdominal cavity. Whether in operating theatres or anatomy classrooms, I've always been stunned by this moment of revelation: that just a few millimetres below the skin lies a glistening clockwork intricacy, the mechanisms that keep us alive. Philip had been dead for a few days, and his viscera were beginning to turn – I had to stifle a gag. But Charlotte was deft and businesslike ('I only wear a mask when there are maggots');* she cut through his rectum and oesophagus, then lifted out all his major abdominal organs – liver, spleen, stomach, intestines – in one piece and onto a plastic tray. Left behind was a hollow, exenterated space. The tray was placed on an examination table for later, and we turned back to the corpse.

The main artery of the leg enters the pelvis just to one side of the bladder. Charlotte squeezed some blood from it, to be sent away for analysis of drugs and toxins. 'From my clinic I usually send urine for toxicology,' I said. 'So do we,' she replied. But where I would send the patient off to the loo with a tiny sample bottle, she made a small hole in the top of the bladder with a knife and sucked some urine out with a syringe.

---

* Forensic pathologists have to be entomologists too: the species of insects found on the body can predict the time of death to a remarkable degree. Edinburgh's pathology department are developing new charts that take into account Scotland's colder climate, and different patterns of insects.

The next step was a delicate dissection of the neck – strikingly gentle after the vigorous opening of the abdomen. There are several layers of muscles in the neck, all of them involved in speech or swallowing. Charlotte peeled away the layers one by one, looking for signs of bruising or haemorrhage – anything that might suggest strangulation. (In anatomy class I was taught the same dissection; like an archaeologist tenderly brushing away earth, the tutor would elevate each strap muscle, eventually reaching the nerve that lies beneath.) There were no signs of bruising or struggle, and the hyoid bone – a C-shaped structure that anchors the tongue – was unbroken. 'No signs of strangling or hanging,' Charlotte said. 'It's always good to document it if you accidently break the hyoid or the larynx in the removal, just in case the body is exhumed for a repeat examination.'

During the frontal cut Charlotte had left the ribs themselves untouched. Now she used secateurs to cut their front ends, all the way up to the collarbones. She cut those too, and lifted away the breastbone to expose the heart and lungs, gleaming in the chest. The heart is held within a tough membrane called the pericardium; Charlotte took care not to pierce it. Then she nimbly cut a U-shaped slice through the floor of the mouth and, because the neck muscles had already been dissected, she was able to pull the tongue, throat, windpipe, lungs and heart away in one piece.

Philip's tongue lay on the dissection tray, slippery and purple, still attached to his throat and gullet. Charlotte began to make neat, precise cuts across its length looking for evidence that it had been bitten or chewed – injuries that might suggest the dead man had suffered an epileptic seizure or a biting struggle just before death. The tongue was normal, so she turned back to the table to deal with the head.

While we'd been busy at the dissection tray, the

mortuary technicians had cut across the top of Philip's scalp from ear to ear, exposing the skull, then peeled the forehead skin forwards over the face. The scalp had also been pulled backwards, and the calvarium – the dome-like part of the skull – removed to reveal the brain. Charlotte scrutinised the membranes and confirmed that there was no evidence of haemorrhage or meningitis, then extracted the brain itself for examination.

Our brains can't bear their own weight out of the skull – that's why they float in briny cerebrospinal fluid, as the foetus floats weightless in the womb. Charlotte placed the brain to one side, creamy and grey, and it sagged into the contours of the tray. Then she stripped back the opalescent meninges of the skull and we peered into the smooth bowl of its base, where the nerves to the face, ears, eyes and tongue enter and exit. 'Have you ever seen an acoustic neuroma?' I asked her – a relatively rare tumour on the nerve running to the ear. 'Oh yes,' she said, 'they're commoner than you think.'

Charlotte pointed out the pearly translucence of the bone overlying the mechanism of the inner ear. 'Can you see it looks purplish – that's blood behind the bone, in the inner ear. You'd think it was a sign of head trauma, but we see that often in drownings.'

'Why?' I asked.

'Gravity,' she said. 'When bodies are carried along in the water they usually float head down, and blood within the veins and arteries begins to leak out of the blood vessels and into the inner ear.'*

There were no fractures in the skull that we could feel. The mortuary technicians packed the space with cotton

---

* Thomas Browne quotes Pliny's insistence that drowned women float prone, and drowned men belly up, *veluti pudori defunctorum parcente natura* – 'nature modestly ordaining this position to conceal the shame of the dead'. He was wrong.

wool and put the calvarium back on. The skin was stitched over as if the brain had never been disturbed.

What was left of Philip lay on the stainless-steel table. All of his major organs had been removed, his abdomen disembowelled, his chest excavated, his ribcage splayed open. Charlotte cradled his head on the now spindle-thin neck, and rocked it gently from side to side, to feel if there were any broken bones. Because his throat and windpipe had been removed it was possible to run a finger along the front of the neck's vertebrae, to check they were all in alignment. Using a knife, she meticulously divided each rib from its neighbours, and moved it back and forth to feel if there were any fractures. The limbs and pelvis were left to themselves: 'There's not much that can kill you in the limbs,' she said. 'And now for the cut-up.'

All the major organs were now laid out in a couple of trays (as a medical student, this was the only part of a post-mortem I'd been allowed to see). Charlotte proceeded methodically, at times with extraordinary finesse. There were moments when she slowed down and scrutinised the tissue in her hands as if struggling to read arcane script. Her examination of the heart, for example, involved making scores of tiny cuts through each of the coronary arteries, looking for any clots that might have caused a heart attack. There were moments too when she moved at speed, such as when she bisected each kidney, or cut the liver into broad slabs to look for cancer and cysts. It was surprising how much of the work she did by feel. 'Some livers are greasy with fat,' she told me. 'Feel here' – she held out a lobe of lung – 'that rubberiness means it's infected, but in the healthier tissue it feels airy and light. Emphysema feels different again; *too* light and airy, like bubble wrap.' There was a creamy yellow plaque on the surface of one of Philip's lungs ('he had probably worked with asbestos'), and Charlotte took a wedge of it away for further examination under the microscope.

Each organ was weighed and carefully catalogued on a whiteboard at one end of the room. 'We're so used to the big hearts of overweight men that it comes as a surprise when we find one of normal size. We start thinking there's something wrong with it.' Charlotte opened Philip's heart to examine its chambers, then looked in the pulmonary arteries for evidence of the jelly-like clots of pulmonary embolism. She guided my fingertips onto the lining of Philip's aorta: it was porridgy, suggesting that he'd had high cholesterol – 'Another big problem among the Scottish population,' she said.

The tongue, throat and larynx had already been examined; now Charlotte looked along the length of the windpipe for tumours, then opened it from behind to look for any obstructions that might have caused choking – there were none. 'There's not much of interest generally in the abdomen,' she said, 'although we do sometimes see tumour seedlings from the bowel, and there are usually plenty of gallstones. See?' She handed me Philip's gall bladder: it felt like a bag of dice.

'Do you ever find anything in the pancreas?' I asked. 'Sometimes tumours, sometimes a big gallstone blocks its exit, but usually not much.' The pancreas generates the enzymes necessary to digest our food, and after death those enzymes are released. As a result, the pancreas auto-digests; the clean contours of the organ transform into liquid as it relents to its constituent parts.*

The long, smooth knives used in autopsies are known as 'brain knives' because their principal use is to cut sections through the brain. Charlotte methodically made sections across the brain's width, starting at the front and

---

* Thomas Browne, *Urne Buriall* I. 'Some, being of the opinion of Thales, that water was the original of all things, thought it most equal to submit unto the principle of putrefaction, and conclude in a moist relentment.'

moving slowly towards the back, each slice about a centime-
tre in depth. She did the same with the cerebellum, cutting
through the connections that sustained his thought and his
identity, hoping to reveal what might have brought about
his death. All the sections were then arranged on a slab so
that Charlotte could take in the whole structure of Philip's
brain in one glance. The brain was partly decomposed, yet
the grey and white matter appeared distinct. There were
no tumours, cysts or evidence of bleeding. Charlotte took
samples from the hippocampus, and part of the cerebellum
(the 'dentate'). 'They're the parts of the brain most sensitive to lack of oxygen,' she said, 'so will show if he was
struggling for air before he died.'

In the brains of people with Parkinson's disease,
pathologists notice an absence of dark tissue towards the
brainstem – the so-called *substantia nigra*. 'With vascular
dementia,' Charlotte said, 'you see little speckles through
the brain, and also in chronic carbon monoxide poisoning.
In multiple sclerosis there are jellied pink areas, where the
nerves' fatty sheaths have broken down.'

All of Philip's organs were placed back in the cavities
of his chest and abdomen, and the wounds were stitched
up until he looked just as he had when he was rolled into
the autopsy suite. The samples Charlotte had taken were
labelled, and would be sent off for further examination.
'The toxicology will go off to the lab too,' she said, 'and
we'll see whether he might have been poisoned. But often
post-mortem is inconclusive. It looks like he had a chest
infection, he doesn't seem to have been assaulted, and there
was no obvious reason for a collapse.'

'So what happens now?'

'The procurator fiscal will take my report into account,
but it's only one part of the evidence.* It's up to her to
decide whether the death was suspicious, not me.'

---

* A Scottish role roughly comparable to that of a coroner.

I knew the routine now. Taking less than an hour with each, Charlotte performed the same sequence of examinations on the other two bodies. When we opened the skull of the woman in her fifties there was blood: she had died of a massive brain haemorrhage, not a heart attack. 'What would the actual mode of death have been?' I asked Charlotte.

'She's likely to have died very quickly,' said Charlotte as she lifted out the woman's brain; 'either a rise in pressure within her cranium because of the haemorrhage would mean that blood couldn't reach and circulate within it, or a brainstem seizure would have terminated her breathing, or even stopped her heart. Look, there's the ruptured one,' she said, gesturing among the small aneurysms that hung like grapes beneath the trellis of her brain. It looked like a tiny, deflated wineskin.

The obese man had indeed choked: when we opened the back of his windpipe, we found incontrovertible lumps of potato. 'And with asphyxiation?' I asked. 'How long would it have taken him to die?'

'He wouldn't have suffered much either,' she said, guessing what I was really asking. 'Forensic studies of asphyxiation have found you lose consciousness within about ten seconds. By twelve or fifteen seconds, seizures begin.' She went on to explain how, at first, blood would have gone on pumping between the man's failing heart and his unconscious brain, until a tipping point was reached – oxygen deprivation would have begun to cause irreversible damage to both organs. I thought back to biochemistry class, and how delicately haemoglobin molecules are calibrated to sustain life. By the time he lost consciousness the man's haemoglobin would have changed from a bright, lava red to a dusky amethyst purple. 'With less oxygen in the blood, there comes a point when heart muscle can't carry on,' Charlotte said; 'it goes into ventricular fibrillation, and the pulse stops.'

Processes all across the body that for decades had maintained life, stitching it together moment to moment – the filtering of blood in the kidneys, the sifting of toxins in the liver, the maintenance of breath in the brainstem – would have slowed to a stop over minutes. 'By three or four minutes into an asphyxiation,' said Charlotte, 'there are no more signs of life.'

WHEN WE HAD FINISHED the last post-mortem I stripped off my apron, gauntlets and gloves, and hosed down my rubber boots. I stood for a long time in the shower, trying to wash off the smell of human dissolution. I had a clinic to go to in the afternoon, and so changed back into trousers, collar and tie, then went back through to Charlotte's office. She was writing up her findings. As I walked in she looked up and smiled.

'So what did you think?' she asked.

'You see so much death,' I said, straightening my tie; 'how does it affect you?'

She paused, and looked back to her papers. 'I don't think about it too much,' she said at last. 'But' – she took a deep breath then smiled again – 'a morning of post-mortems, it always makes me want to celebrate being alive.'

On the main road outside, a dead rat had been flattened by traffic; a crow was picking at its remains. I got on my bike and pedalled half a mile to my own clinic.

All that afternoon, and for a couple of months afterwards, after-images from the post-mortem room flashed through my memory. 'Autopsy' means 'to see for oneself' – it felt as if a veil had been pulled aside, and a terrible fragility revealed. I'd be talking with a patient then suddenly imagine them laid out on the mortuary slab, their eyes glazed, their blood cold and dark. Those moments were shocking, but also somehow motivating. Medicine is in some ways the art of postponing death, and I returned to my work with new energy.

24

Transformations

How long can this go on? But let us by all means extend the scope of our charts.

Annie Dillard, Holy the Firm

JUST UNDER FOUR THOUSAND people are registered with my medical practice, and at times their difficulties seem to flow like a torrent through the clinic. But I'm conscious that my colleagues and I catch only the briefest glimpse of their lives, our consultations just momentary eddies in a vast tide of human life. Across the span of a morning clinic I might arrange an admission to a hospice, mitigate a storm of anxiety, explore a worrying discomfort, medicate a feverish baby, adjust some antipsychotics, assess a healing fracture. I might celebrate a remission of cancer, or commiserate over its diagnosis; voice congratulations on the safe birth of a baby, and condolences over the death of a spouse. Some of the work is modest and routine, some is urgent and dramatic, most of it is rewarding and worthwhile. At its best, medicine invokes and influences human change, and the possibility of change means hope.

There's a quick walk I can take from my medical office up to an outcrop of cliffs overlooking Edinburgh's city centre. The cliffs are known as 'Salisbury Crags', and the land around them has long been a protected royal park. The view from them always grants perspective. Their rock is of cooled magma, thrust out more than three hundred million years ago by the pleating and wrenching of the earth's crust. Scotland lay nearer the equator then, and the local bedrock – an uplifted ocean floor – was already ancient. You can still see the step between the softer sandstone base and the hard magma intrusion of the cliffs. For centuries, the city streets were cobbled with the durable rocks of Salisbury Crags.

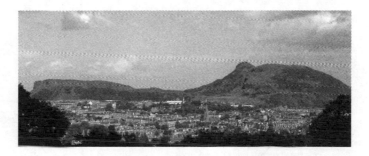

In the 1780s a local physician, chemist and farmer called James Hutton examined the crags, and realised what they testified: the earth's surface was not static, but slowly churning. He delivered a paper to the Royal Society of Edinburgh arguing that the sandstone beneath the crags had been created 'in the unfathomable regions of the sea', before rising up to become land. He was resurrecting an ancient idea: in the *Metamorphoses*, Ovid described land and sea caught in cycles of transformation, one into another: 'I have seen what once was solid earth now changed into sea,' Ovid wrote, 'and lands created out of what once was ocean.' Hutton summoned a vision of eternal, universal flux: 'we find no vestige of a beginning – no prospect of an end.'

From my habitual perch on the clifftop I can see my practice area laid out below me like a living map. Patches of cloud shadow and light move over the face of the city, merging and dividing. The fluid lives of my patients are reflected in the street movements of cars and pedestrians. From up there I can see the old medical school and the adjacent park of elm and cherry trees, where I first had a revelation of the dynamism and elegance of biochemistry. There's the tree where Gary Hobbes fell, convinced he'd become a cat, as well as the housing scheme where Hannah Mollier conceived three pregnancies, and Harry Alkman injected himself with bodybuilding drugs. There are the bars and tattoo parlours my patients frequent; their apartments, offices and college halls. To the north, there's the morgue, to the south, the crematorium, and between them, the green baize of several burial grounds. There's the rehabilitation hospital I refer to for prosthetics, and the sexual health centre with its menopause and gender clinics. Off to the west there's the hill of Craiglockhart, where W. H. R. Rivers sought the redemption of war memories; closer by there's the dementia centre run by his heirs. Visible too is a research institute where, even now, genetic mutations that were millennia in evolution are being replicated in minutes. Our species has the power now to transform its own DNA – an ability that may yet prove a curse, or a consolation.

Ovid's *Metamorphoses* ends on a note of optimism. It conjures a vision of the citizens of Rome, out on the streets to receive the god of medicine who has journeyed from Greece to save the city from a pestilence. The god arrives in the form of a snake, symbol of transformation and renewal; it winds through the streets before coming to rest on an island that divides the flow of the river Tiber. Once there, the god 'resumed his divine appearance, put an end to the citizens' distress, and brought health to the city by his coming'. The final lines see Julius Caesar deified, hoisted to heaven, and transformed into a star. Ovid proclaims that the magnificence of his own poem has rendered him immortal. But no one is immortal, nothing is eternal, everything is in flux – even the stars.

This world always was, is, and will be an ever-living Fire, with measures of it kindling, and measures going out … it rests by changing.

Heraclitus, *Fragments* 30, 84

Gratitude

TWENTY YEARS OF REMEMBERED clinical encounters are the inspiration for this book, and the people to whom I'm most grateful are my patients. The requirement to honour their confidentiality means that they must go unthanked individually. I'm also thankful to Andrew Franklin, Cecily Gayford and Penny Daniel of Profile, and Kirty Topiwala of the Wellcome Collection, for their trust, support and editorial talent. Susanne Hillen copy-edited the manuscript beautifully. A bouquet of gratitude too for Jenny Brown – the only literary agent I know who offers babysitting.

I'm grateful to Lee Illis for his insights into porphyria and lycanthropy, and Genevieve Lively for permitting me to quote from her book on Ovid. Some ideas in 'Conception' were inspired by Thomas Laqueur's 1986 essay 'Orgasm, generation, and the politics of reproductive biology'. Carrie Vout of Cambridge University kept me right with Ovid, and with Hercules. Douglas Cairns kept me right with Heraclitus and with Nicander. 'Bodybuilding' couldn't have been written without Sven Lindqvist's *Bench Press*. Claire Preston's work on Thomas Browne was instrumental in the writing of 'Scalp'. Malcolm MacCallum at the University of Edinburgh has given enormously of his time and energy in supporting my research for this book. Thomas Morris's *The Matter of the Heart* helped me in writing 'Birth' and Marina Warner guided me through European and Near Eastern rejuvenation myths. I gratefully acknowledge the contribution to 'Anorexia' of Katy Waldman's brilliant *Slate* essay 'There once was a girl'. For 'Hallucination', I gratefully thank Theresa Kiyota and acknowledge the influence of Paul and John Lysaker's 2010 'Schizophrenia and alterations in self-experience'. Thomas Williams of the University of Edinburgh and Louise Bath of Edinburgh's Royal Hospital for Sick Children both gave generously of their time and their thoughts in helping me with 'Puberty' and 'Gigantism', as did James Hall and Iain McClure. For 'Pregnancy', I'm grateful to Chitra Ramaswamy for allowing me to quote from her book *Expecting*. Maggie Nelson graciously permitted me to quote from *The Argonauts*, and Elan Anthony to quote his views on detransitioning. I'm grateful to Professor Dick Swaab for confirming with me the details of the post-mortem studies quoted in 'Gender'. Diane Mickley permitted me to quote her views on anorexia. Thanks are due to Professor Jo Arendt for supervising my Masters thesis on circadian clocks in Antarctica – some of the material in 'Jetlag' is thanks to her. James Kern generously gave permission to quote his words on the redemption of unwanted tattoos. I'm grateful to Stephen Owens, Kalilu Sanneh and Conor Doherty, for welcoming me to Keneba in the Gambia. Thanks to Ailsa Gebbie for inviting me to her menopause clinic in Edinburgh, and to the late Ursula Le Guin, Louise Foxcroft, Germaine Greer and Iona Heath, for giving me permission to reproduce their reflections on the menopause, published and unpublished. Sergio Bestente introduced me to Martha Feldman's book *The Castrato* and is a fine editor and friend; thanks to the estate of Anatole Broyard for giving permission to quote from his collection of essays. Penguin Books granted kind permission to quote from *Metamorphosis* by Ovid. trans. Mary M. Innes. Copyright © Mary M. Innes, 1995. Andrew Gannon, Olivia Giles and Jamie Andrew all gave generously of their time in helping me understand more about their use of, and work with, prosthetic limbs. Professor Richard

Morris of the University of Edinburgh shared his ideas on memory and brain injury. Thanks to Karen Edgar in New York, and the estate of Alexander Luria in Moscow, for permitting me to quote Luria's letter to Oliver Sacks, previously published in *The Man Who Mistook His Wife for a Hat*. Damien Hirst kindly granted permission to quote his comments to *The Telegraph* on death and vigour. David Farrier and Peter Dorward read an early version of the typescript and gave insightful comments.

An early version of 'Gender' first appeared in *The New Republic* in November 2015; the writing of it, with the help of Sarah Kennedy and Jennifer Whyte, set me off on a journey into human transformation. I'm grateful to the editors for permitting elements of it to be reproduced here, and to Laura Marsh and Emma Foehringer Merchant for their skill in editing it. Earlier versions of 'Werewolves' and 'Death' first appeared in the *London Review of Books*; I'm grateful to Mary-Kay Wilmers for permitting them to be reproduced here, and Paul Myerscough for editing them so attentively. Some of the material in 'Sleep' was unearthed during research for my essay 'Cerebral Hygiene', published in the *London Review of Books*, and material on the networks of synaptic plasticity reproduced in 'Memory' was courtesy of research for my piece on Santiago Ramón y Cajal, 'In The Flower Garden of the Brain' in the *New York Review of Books*.

My colleagues at Dalkeith Road Medical Practice are incomparable: thanks to Teresa Quinn, Fiona Wright, Ishbel White, Janis Blair, Geraldine Fraser, Pearl Ferguson, Jenna Pemberton, Lynsay McDonald, Sharon Lawson, and Nicola Gray.

My final thanks are to Esa, for all the changes so far through the seasons of our lives.

Notes on Sources

1. Transformations
p. 3. Ovid, *Metamorphoses*, Book XV, lines 169–75.

2. Werewolves: Agitation at the Full Moon
p. 6. Genevieve Liveley, *Ovid's 'Metamorphoses'* (London: Continuum Books, 2011), p. 22.

p. 6. M. D. Angus, 'The rejection of two explanations of belief in a lunar influence on behavior', in D. E. Vance, ed., 'Belief in lunar effects on human behavior', *Psychological Reports*, 76 (1995), p. 32.

p. 7. Charles Raison, Haven Klein and Morgan Steckler, 'The moon and madness reconsidered', *The Journal of Affective Disorders* vol. 53, no. 1, April 1999, pp. 99–106.

p. 7. Jean-Étienne Esquirol, *Mental Maladies, A Treatise On Insanity* (Philadelphia: Lea and Blanchard, 1845, translated from the French), pp. 32–33.

p. 10. In 1969 it was proposed that King George III (reigned 1760–1820) had a variant of porphyria, but this has since been debunked as unlikely. See I. Macalpine and R. Hunter, *George III and the Mad Business* (London: Penguin Press, 1969).

p. 10. L. Illis, 'On porphyria and the aetiology of werwolves', *Proceedings of the Royal Society of Medicine* vol. 57, 1964, pp. 23–26.

p. 11. *Encyclopaedia Metropolitana*, Edward Smedley, Hugh James Rose and Henry John Rose, eds (London: B. Fellowes et al., 1845), p. 618.

p. 12. Paul M. C. Forbes Irving, *Metamorphosis in Greek Myths* (Oxford: Clarendon Press, 1990).

p. 12. *The History of the World, Commonly Called the Natural History of C. Plinius Secundus, or Pliny* (New York: McGraw-Hill, 1964), Book VIII, chapter 22, p. 65.

p. 12. Virgil, *Eclogues* VI, 'The Song of Silenus'.

p. 12. Daniel 4:33.

p. 12. C. G. Jung, *Collected Works*, vol. 17 (London: Routledge and Kegan Paul, 1954). Jung's story is an interesting reversal of the legend of Dante Alighieri's mother, who famously dreamed while pregnant that her unborn son would transform into a peacock.

p. 14. See Forbes Irving, *Metamorphosis in Greek Myths*.

p. 15. Paul E. Keck, Harrison G. Pope, James I. Hudson, Susan L. McElroy and Aaron R. Kulick, 'Lycanthropy: alive and well in the twentieth century', *Psychological Medicine* vol. 18, no. 1, 1988, pp. 113–20.

3. Conception: The First and Second Reason for Existing

p. 18. Quoted in Sarah Bakewell, *How to Live: A Life of Montaigne in One Question and Twenty Attempts at an Answer* (London: Random House, 2011), p. 20.

p. 18. Notebook from 1504: 'Questo scriver si distintamente del nibbio par che sia mio destino, perchè nella prima ricordatione della mia infantia e' mi parea che, essendo io in culla, un nibbio venisse a me e mi aprissi la bocca colla sua coda e molte volte mi percuotesse colla sua coda dentro alle labbra.' Translated in Meyer Shapiro's paper 'Leonardo and Freud – An art historical study', *Journal of the History of Ideas* vol. 17, no. 2, April 1956, pp. 47–78: 'This writing distinctly about the vulture seems to be my destiny, because among the first recollections of my infancy it seemed to me that as I lay in my cradle a vulture came to me and opened my mouth with its tail and struck me many times with its tail inside my lips.'

p. 18. Pliny's *Natural History*: 'It seems that this bird by the movements of its tail taught the art of steermanship, nature demonstrating in the sky what was required in the deep.'

p. 20. In English it was published another twenty years later, in 1545, as *The Byrth of Mankynde*.

p. 20. Cited in V. C. Medvei, *A History of Endocrinology* (Lancaster and Hingham, Massachusetts: MTP Press, 1982), p. 357; Albrecht von Haller, *Physiology: Being a Course of Lectures*, vol. 2 (1754), paragraphs 823–26, pp. 301–303.

p. 20. Q. U. Newell et al., 'The time of ovulation in the menstrual cycle as checked by the recovery of ova from the Fallopian tubes', *American Journal of Obstetrics and Gynecology*, vol. 19, February 1930, pp. 180–85; George W. Corner, 'Our knowledge of the menstrual cycle, 1910–1950', *The Lancet* vol. 240, no. 6661, 28 April 1951, pp. 919–23.

p. 25. Robert Latou Dickinson, *Human Sex Anatomy* (Baltimore: The Wilton and Williams Company, 1933). Dickinson lists dozens of German sources, including Litzmann (1846), Kristeller (1871), Wernich (1872) and Kisch (1895).

p. 26. Dickinson, *Human Sex Anatomy*, p. vii.

p. 26. Ibid., p. 84.

p. 26. Ibid., p. 109.

p. 26. 'Magnetic resonance imaging of male and female genitals during coitus and female sexual arousal', in *BMJ* vol. 319, 1999, pp. 596–600.

4. Sleep: The Chamber of Dreams

p. 32. Fabian Guénolé, Geoffrey Marcaggi and Jean-Marc Baleyte, 'Do dreams really guard sleep? Evidence for and against Freud's theory of the basic function of dreaming', *Frontiers in Psychology* vol. 4, no. 17, 2013.

p. 34. As translated by Henry Riley, London, 1893.

p. 34. *The Epic of Gilgamesh*, Book III: 'then he transformed me so that my arms became wings covered with feathers'.

p. 37. Richard Stephenson and Vern Lewis, 'Behavioural evidence for a sleep-like quiescent state in a pulmonate mollusc, *Lymnaea stagnalis* (Linnaeus)', *Journal of Experimental Biology* vol. 214, 2011 pp. 747–56.

p. 37. *The Interpretation of Dreams, digested into five books by that ancient and excellent philosopher, Artemidorus*, Robert Wood, trans. (London, 1644).

5. Bodybuilding: Unhelmed by Fury

p. 39. Quoted by Xenophon in *Memorabilia*, Book II, chapter
1, in E. C. Marchant, ed., *Xenophon 4* (Cambridge,
Massachusetts: Harvard University Press; London: William
Heinemann, Ltd, 1923).

p. 42. The trophy turned out to be brass thinly plated in gold.
See Andrew Lycett, *Conan Doyle: The Man Who Created
Sherlock Holmes* (London: Phoenix Books, 2008), p. 284.

p. 42. For a deeper exploration of these themes, see Maria
Wyke, 'Herculean muscle!: The classicizing rhetoric of
bodybuilding', *Journal of Humanities and the Classics*,
Third Series, vol. 4, no. 3, Winter, 1997, pp. 51–79.

p. 43. *Arnold Schwarzenegger: The Education of a Bodybuilder*
(London: Sphere Books, 1979), pp. 14–15.

p. 43. Psychiatrists have found a preponderance of 'pathological
narcissism' among weightlifters, particularly those who use
steroids. See J. H. Porcerelli and B. A. Sandler, 'Narcissism
and empathy in steroid users', *American Journal of
Psychiatry* vol. 152, no. 11, 1995, pp. 1672–74.

p. 44. Arnold Schwarzenegger, *Encyclopedia of Modern
Bodybuilding* (London: Michael Joseph, 1987), p. 725.

p. 45. *The Complete Greek Drama Volume One*, Whitney J.
Oates and Eugene O'Neill Jr, eds, with plays by Euripides
translated by E. P. Coleridge (New York: Random House,
1938).

p. 47. See, for example, Brian Corrigan, 'Anabolic steroids and the
mind', *Medical Journal of Australia* vol. 165, 1996, pp.
222–26.

p. 47. Helen Keane, 'Diagnosing the male steroid user: drug use,
body image and disordered masculinity', *Health* vol. 9,
no. 2, 2005, pp. 89–208.

6. Scalp: Of Horns, Terror and Glory

p. 53. *Totem and Taboo*, in *The Standard Edition of the Complete
Psychological Works of Sigmund Freud*, vol. XIII (London:
Hogarth Press, 1955), p. 213.

p. 53. 'Equally amazed was Cipus, the Republican general, when he
looked at himself in the waters of the river: for he saw horns
sprouting from his brow.' Ovid, *Metamorphoses*, Mary

Innes, trans. (London: Penguin Classics, 1955), Book XV, line 560.

p. 53. Sir Thomas Browne, *Selected Writings*, Claire Preston, ed. (Manchester: Carcanet Press, 1995), *Pseudodoxia Epidemica*, p. 69.

p. 54. Leon J. Saul, MD and Clarence Bernstein Jr, MD, 'Emotional settings of some attacks of Urticaria', *Psychosomatic Medicine* vol. 3, no. 3, October 1941, pp. 49–69.

p. 54. L. Landois, 'Das plötzliche Ergrauen der Haupthaare', *Archiv fur pathologische Anatomie und Physiologie* vol. 35, 1866, p. 575.

p. 55. For an irreverent but scholarly appreciation of the phenomenon, see J. E. Jelinek's review 'Sudden whitening of the hair', presented at a meeting of the Section on Historical Medicine of the New York Academy of Medicine, 22 March 1972.

p. 55. Byron recognised that the phenomenon didn't happen overnight, when he wrote of Sforza in *The Prisoner of Chillon*, as quoted at the beginning of this chapter: 'My hair is grey/ but not with years / Nor grew it white / In a single night / As men's have grown from sudden fears.'

p. 55. Stefan Zweig, *Mary Stuart* (London: Pushkin Press, 2010); Wordsworth's 'Lament for Mary Queen of Scots': 'Those shocks of passion can prepare / That kill the bloom before its time / And blanch, without the owner's crime / The most resplendent hair.'

7. Birth: Reshaping the Heart

p. 61. M. S. Sutton, A. Groves and A. MacNeill et al., 'Assessment of changes in blood flow through the lungs and foramen ovale in the normal human fetus with gestational age: a prospective Doppler echocardiographic study', *Heart* vol. 71, 1994, pp. 232–37.

p. 61. D. C. Little et al., 'Patent ductus arteriosus in micropreemies and full-term infants: The relative merits of surgical ligation versus indomethacin treatment', *Journal of Pediatric Surgery* vol. 38, no. 3, 2003, pp. 492–96.

p. 62. Quoted in Charles Harris, *The Heart and the Vascular System in Ancient Greek Medicine: From Alcmaeon to Galen* (Oxford: Clarendon Press, 1973), pp. 294–95.

p. 63. J. E. Dice and J. Bhatia, 'Patent ductus arteriosus: An overview', *The Journal of Pediatric Pharmacology and Therapeutics* vol. 12, no. 3, July–September 2007, pp. 138–46.

p. 66. Robert E. Gross, MD, 'Surgical management of the patent ductus arteriosus with summary of four surgically treated cases', *Annals of Surgery* vol. 110, no. 3, 1939, pp. 321–56.

8. Rejuvenation: An Alchemy of Youth and Beauty

p. 69. A. S. F. Gow and A. F. Scholfield, *Nicander: The Poems and Poetical Fragments* (Cambridge: Cambridge University Press, 1953), pp. 42–45. This is fragment 62.

p. 69. Mikhail Bulgakov, *The Master and Margarita*, Michael Glenny, trans. (London: Vintage Classics, 2010).

p. 75. *Chou-i ts'an t'ung ch'i.*

9. Tattooing: The Art of Transformation

p. 83. Arthur Conan Doyle, *The Red-Headed League*, p. 3.

p. 84. See Donaghy's poem 'Liverpool' in *Errata* (Oxford: Oxford University Press, 1993).

p. 84. See Ronald Scutt and Christopher Gotch, *Skin Deep* (London: Peter Davies Ltd, 1974).

p. 88. See Chee-Leok Goh and Stephanie G. Ho, 'Lasers for tattoo removal', in K. Lahiri, A. De and A. Sarda, *Textbook of Lasers in Dermatology* (London: J. P. Medical Ltd, 2016).

10. Anorexia: The Enchantment of Control

p. 90. Diane Mickley, MD, Wilkins Center for Eating Disorders, Greenwich, Connecticut; personal communication.

p. 92. Rudolph Bell, *Holy Anorexia* (Chicago: University of Chicago Press, 1985).

p. 92. L. K. Oyewumi and S. S. Kazarian, 'Abnormal eating attitudes among a group of Nigerian youths: II. Anorexic behaviour', *East African Medical Journal* vol. 69, 1992, pp. 67–69.

p. 92. S. Lee, T. Ho and I.. Hsu, 'Fat phobic and non-fat phobic anorexia nervosa: a comparative study of 70 Chinese patients in Hong Kong', *Psychological Medicine* vol. 23, 1993, pp. 99–1017.

p. 92. D. Wassenaar, D. le Grange and J. Winship et al. 'The prevalence of eating disorder pathology in a cross-ethnic population of female students in South Africa', *European Eating Disorders Review* vol. 8, 2000, pp. 25–36.

p. 92. M. Husni, N. Koye and J. Haggarty, 'Severe anorexia in an Amish Mennonite teenager', *The Canadian Journal of Psychiatry* vol. 46, no. 2, 2001, p. 183.

p. 92. There are an abundance of these, but in terms of essay-length pieces I can recommend Carrie Arnold's 'A grown-up approach to treating anorexia', published online by Mosaic Science on 29 March 2016 (mosaicscience.com).

p. 96. Charles Lasègue, 'On Hysterical Anorexia', 1873.

p. 96. 'There once was a girl – against the false narratives of anorexia', *Slate*, December 2015 cover story.

11. Hallucination: A Sphere of Devils

p. 100. Eugen Bleuler, *Dementia Praecox, or the Group of Schizophrenias*, Joseph Zinkin, trans. (New York: International Universities Press, 1950), p. 143.

p. 101. D. T. Suzuki, in the preface to R. H. Blyth, *Zen and Zen Classics Volume Four 'Mumonkan'* (Tokyo: Hokusaido Press, 1966).

p. 101. See Koji Sato's illuminating paper, 'D. T. Suzuki, Zen and LSD 25', *Psychologia* vol. 10, 1967, pp. 129–32.

p. 102. Johann M. Faber, *Strychnomania explicans strychni manici antiquorum, vel solani furiosi recentiorum, historiae monumentum, indolis nocumentum, antidoti documentum*, 1677.

p. 106. R. D. Laing, *The Divided Self* (New York: Penguin Books, 1978), p. 151.

p. 106. Giovanni Stanghellini, *Disembodied Spirits and Deanimated Bodies* (Oxford: Oxford University Press, 2004), p. 126.

12. Puberty: Suddenly Accelerated Youth

p. 112. J. M. Tanner, *Growth at Adolescence 2nd Edn* (Oxford: Blackwell, 1962), p. 240.

p. 112. W. A. Marshall and J. M. Tanner, 'Variation in the pattern of pubertal changes in girls', *Archives of Disease in Childhood* vol. 44, 1969, p. 291; and W. A. Marshall and J. M. Tanner, 'Variation in the pattern of pubertal changes in boys', *Archives of Disease in Childhood* vol. 45, 1970, p. 13.

p. 114. See James S. Chisholm et al., 'Early stress predicts age at menarche and first birth, adult attachment, and expected lifespan', *Human Nature* vol. 16, no. 3, 2005, pp. 233–65.

p. 116. Tanner, *Growth at Adolescence* (1962), p. 220, referencing L. K. Frank, R. Harrison, E. Hellersberg, K. Machover and M. Steiner, 'Personality development in adolescent girls', *Monographs of the Society for Research in Child Development* vol. 16, 1951, p. 316.

p. 118. J. M. Siegel et al., 'Body image, perceived pubertal timing, and adolescent mental health', *Journal of Adolescent Health* vol. 25, no. 2, August 1999, pp. 55–65.

p. 118. C. Berge, 'Heterochronic processes in human evolution: An ontogenetic analysis of the hominid pelvis', *American Journal of Physical Anthropology* vol. 105, no. 4, pp. 41–59.

13. Pregnancy: The Most Meticulous Work

p. 119. Hogarth's personal correspondence, quoted in John L. Thornton and Patricia C. Want, 'William Hunter (1718–1783) and his contributions to obstetrics', *British Journal of Obstetrics and Gynaecology* vol. 90, September 1983, pp. 787–94.

p. 119. I. Donald, J. Macvicar and T. G. Brown, 'The investigation of abdominal masses by pulsed ultrasound', *Lancet* vol. 271, no. 7032, 7 June 1958, pp. 188–95.

p. 122. Chitra Ramaswamy, *Expecting: The Inner Life of Pregnancy* (Salford: Saraband, 2006), p. 101.

p. 122. Ibid., p. 67.

p. 126. Peter M. Dunn, 'Leonardo da Vinci (1452–1519) and reproductive anatomy', *BMJ* vol. 77, no. 3, November 1997.

p. 126. From da Vinci's notebooks, quoted in Antonio J. Ferreira, 'Emotional factors in prenatal environment: A review', *Journal of Nervous and Mental Disease* vol. 141, no. 1, July 1965, pp. 108–18.

p. 127. Virgina Woolf, *Orlando: A Biography* (Oxford: Oxford University Press, 2014), p. 136.

p. 127. Margaret Atwood, *The Handmaid's Tale* (London: Vintage, 2016), p. 42 and p. 43.

p. 127. Chitra Ramaswamy, *Expecting*, p. 70.

p. 128. J. van Rymsdyk and A. van Rymsdyk, *Museum Britannicum* (London: Moore, 1778), p. 83.

p. 129. Notes from an exhibition: 'Contributions of the Hunter brothers to our understanding of reproduction: An exhibition from the University Library's collections', Special Collections department, Glasgow University Library 16 July–30 September 1992.

p. 129. See Margaret Hunt, *Women in Eighteenth-Century Europe* (London: Routledge, 2009), p. 100.

p. 129. *An anatomical description of the human gravid uterus and its contents, by the Late William Hunter, MD* (London: printed for J. Johnson, and G. Nicol, 1794).

14. Gigantism: Two Giants of Turin

p. 133. *Selected Letters of Friedrich Nietzsche*, Christopher Middleton, trans. (Indianapolis: Hackete, 1996), p. 296.

p. 133. *Selected Letters of Friedrich Nietzsche*, Christopher Middleton, trans., letter to Peter Gast, 30 October 1888, p. 318.

p. 135. Friedrich Nietzsche, *Ecce Homo* (London: Macmillan, 1911), p. 120.

p. 135. Friedrich Nietzsche, *Philosophy in the Tragic Age of the Greeks*, Marianne Cowan, trans. (Washington, DC: Regnery Publishing, 1996), p. 3.

p. 136. John of Salisbury: 'Bernard of Chartres used to compare us to [puny] dwarfs perched on the shoulders of giants', *Metalogicon* (1159), quoted in *The Metalogicon of John of Salisbury: A Twelfth-Century Defense of the Verbal and Logical Arts of the Trivium*, Daniel D. McGarry, trans. (Westport, Connecticut: Greenwood Press, 1982).

p. 137. At least according to Miroslav Holub, the Czech poet and immunologist. See 'The intimate life of nude mice', in *The Dimension of the Present Moment and Other Essays* (London: Faber and Faber, 1990), p. 39.

p. 138. See J. T. Lie and S. J. Grossman, 'Pathology of the heart in acromegaly: anatomic findings in 27 autopsied patients', *American Heart Journal* vol. 100, no. 1, 1980, pp. 1–52.

p. 138. Quoted in Walter Kaufmann, *Nietzsche: Philosopher, Psychologist, Antichrist* (Princeton: Princeton University Press, 1974), p. 46.

p. 139. Stephen Hall, *Size Matters* (Boston: Houghton Mifflin, 2006), p. 177.

p. 141. 'That to philosophize is to learn to die', in *The Complete Essays of Montaigne*, Donald Frame, trans. (Palo Alto, California: Stanford University Press, 1965), p. 67.

p. 141. *The Complete Works of Montaigne*, Donald Frame, trans. (Palo Alta, California: Stanford University Press, 1957), pp. 69–70.

15. Gender: The Two Lives of Tiresias

p. 152. F. Abraham, 'Genitalumwandlungen an zwei männlichen Transvestiten', *Zeitschrift für Sexualwissenschaft und Sexualpolitik* vol. 18, 1931, pp. 23–26, translated and republished as 'Genital reassignment on two male transvestites', *International Journal of Transgenderism* vol. 2, no. 1, January–March 1998.

p. 153. Burou is quoted on the website, Trans Media Watch.

p. 154. This was suggested in a 1995 paper in *Nature*: J.-N. Zhou, M. A. Hofman, L. J. Gooren and D. F. Swaab, 'A sex difference in the human brain and its relation to transsexuality', *Nature* vol. 378, pp. 68–70. A later study from California disputed the chain of causation, arguing that the brain structure changed slowly over time due to a change in behaviour.

p. 155. Maggie Nelson, *The Argonauts* (London: Melville Press, 2016), pp. 65, 103.

p. 155. *The Guardian*, 'Family' section, 16 September 2017, p. 5.

16. Jetlag: The Brain that Holds the Sky

p. 161. Aarti Jagannath et al., 'The CRTC1-SIK1 pathway regulates entrainment of the circadian clock', *Cell* vol. 154, no. 5, 29 August 2013, pp. 100–111.

p. 162. Gavin Francis et al., 'Sleep during the Antarctic winter: Preliminary observations on changing the spectral composition of artificial light', *Journal of Sleep Research* vol. 17, 2008, pp. 54–60.

17. Bonesetting: An Algebra of Healing

p. 172. See Michael Marmot, *Status Syndrome* (London: Bloomsbury, 2015).

18. Menopause: Third Face of the Goddess

p. 176. 'The 30 or 35 years of menstrual life, i.e. from puberty to menopause', 'Ovarian Tumours', 1872, cited in the *Shorter Oxford English Dictionary*.

p. 177. Respectively, 'Georgius Castriotus ... died upon this day in his climactericall year 63' in Lloyd's *Dial Daies*; and 'the climacteric effacement of the breast' in Bryant's *Practical Surgery*, as cited in the OED.

p. 177. Louise Foxcroft, *Hot Flushes, Cold Science: A History of the Menopause* (London: Granta, 2009), from the introduction.

p. 177. Roy Porter, *The Greatest Benefit to Mankind: A Medical History of Humanity* (London: HarperCollins, 1999), pp. 706–7.

p. 178. Nancy Datan, 'Aging into transitions: Cross-cultural perspectives on women at midlife', in *The Meanings of Menopause*, Ruth Formanek, ed. (Hillsdale, New Jersey: The Analytic Press, 1990), pp. 117–31.

p. 180. Eleanor Mann et al., 'Cognitive behavioural treatment for women who have menopausal symptoms after breast cancer treatment (MENOS 1): a randomised controlled trial', *The Lancet Oncology* vol. 13, no. 3, March 2012, pp. 309–18.

p. 181. Germaine Greer, *The Change: Women, Ageing and the Menopause* (London: Hamish Hamilton, 1991), p. 124.

p. 182. Carol Gilligan, *In a Different Voice: Psychological Theory and Women's Development* (Cambridge, Massachusetts: Harvard University Press, 1982), p. 171.

p. 182. Ursula K. Le Guin, 'The Space Crone', in *Dancing at the Edge of the World* (New York: Grove Press, 1989).

19. Castration: Hope, Love and Sacrifice

p. 184. Quoted in Anatole Broyard, 'Reading and writing; Life before death', *New York Times*, 6 June 1982.

p. 187. Martha Feldman, *The Castrato* (Oakland, California: University of California Press, 2015), p. 14.

p. 189. Anatole Broyard, *Intoxicated by my Illness* (New York: Fawcett Columbine, 1992), p. 22.

p. 189. Ibid.

p. 189. Ibid., p. 36.

p. 189. Ibid., p. 40.

p. 189. Ibid., p. 26.

p. 191. Ibid., p. 27.

p. 193. Brian Steidle and Gretchen Wallace, *The Devil Came on Horseback: Bearing Witness to the Genocide in Darfur* (New York: Perseus Books, 2007), p. 88.

p. 193. Sir Thomas Browne, *Selected Writings*, Claire Preston, ed., *Pseudodoxia Epidemica*.

p. 193. Lucretius, *The Nature of Things* (London: Penguin Classics, 2007), Book VI, line 1207.

p. 194. Matthew 19:12.

20. Laughter: Some Eminency in Ourselves

p. 197. M. Demir, 'Effects of laughter therapy on anxiety, stress, depression and quality of life in cancer patients', *The Journal of Cancer Science & Therapy* vol. 7, 2015, pp. 272–73.

p. 197. See R. Provine, *Laughter: A Scientific Investigation* (London: Penguin, 2000).

p. 198. Charles Darwin, *On the Expression of Emotion in Man and Animals* (London: John Murray, 1872), p. 343.

p. 199. *Hippocratic Writings*, G. Lloyd, ed. (London: Penguin Classics, 1983), 'Epidemics, Book III'.

p. 200. Charles Darwin, *On the Expression of Emotion in Man and Animals*, p. 342.

p. 200. P. C. Jacob and R. P. Chand, 'Pathological laughter following intravenous sodium valproate', *Canadian Journal of Neurological Sciences* vol. 25, 1998, pp. 252–53.

p. 200. J. Parvizi et al., 'Pathological laughter and crying: A link to the cerebellum', *Brain* vol. 124, no. 9, 2001, pp. 1708–719.

p. 200. F. A. Gondim, B. J. Parks and S. Cruz-Flores, '"Fou rire prodromique" as the presentation of pontine ischaemia secondary to vertebrobasilar stenosis', *Journal of Neurology, Neurosurgery, and Psychiatry* vol. 71, 2001, pp. 802–804.

p. 201. Basil Bunting, *Briggflatts* (Hexham: Bloodaxe Books, 2009).

21. Prosthetics: Humanity 2.0

p. 202. The sixth book of Ovid's *Metamorphoses*, verse 401.

p. 209. Some studies have found that calamitous events, such as disabling accidents, or longed-for events, such as winning the lottery, have little long-term effect on levels of personal happiness. See P. Brickman, D. Coates and R. Janoff-Bulman, 'Lottery winners and accident victims: Is happiness relative?', *The Journal of Personality and Social Psychology* vol. 36, 1978, pp. 917–27.

22. Memory: Palaces of Forgetting

p. 213. William James, *The Principles of Psychology*, authorised edn, vol. 1 (New York: Henry Holt, 1890; repr., New York: Dover, 1950), pp. 680–81.

p. 218. See Schrödinger's *Nature and the Greeks*, first published in 1954, which attempted to bridge an understanding gap between religion and modern science.

p. 218. Erwin Schrödinger, *What is Life? & Mind and Matter* (Cambridge: Cambridge University Press, 1967), Epilogue, p. 96.

p. 218. Schrödinger, 'Oneness of Mind' in *What is Life? & Mind and Matter* (Cambridge: Cambridge University Press, 1967), p. 145.

p. 218. Schrödinger, *What is Life? & Mind and Matter*, p. 147.

p. 218. Homer's *The Odyssey*, D. C. H. Rieu, ed. (London: Penguin Classics, 2003), Book VIII, line 487.

p. 221. Janine M. Cooper et al., 'Neonatal hypoxia, hippocampal atrophy, and memory impairment: Evidence of a causal sequence', *Cerebral Cortex* vol. 25, no. 6, 1 June 2015, pp. 469–76.

p. 221. Susan M. Ravizza et al., 'Cerebellar damage produces selective deficits in verbal working memory', *Brain* vol. 129, no. 2, February 2006, pp. 306–20.

p. 223. *The History of the World, Commonly Called the Natural History of C. Plinius Secundus, or Pliny* (New York: McGraw-Hill, 1964), Book VII, chapter 24.

p. 226. W. H. R. Rivers, 'An address on the repression of war experience', *The Lancet* vol. 191, no. 4927, 2 February 1918, p. 173.

p. 227. *The Muse in Arms*, E. B. Osborn, ed. (London: John Murray, 1917).

23. Death: The Celebration of Life

p. 229. 'Damien Hirst: "We're here for a good time, not a long time"', interview with Alastair Sooke, *Daily Telegraph*, 8 January 2011.

p. 238. See Anny Sauvageau et al., 'Agonal sequences in 14 filmed hangings with comments on the role of the type of suspension, ischemic habituation, and ethanol intoxication on the timing of agonal responses', *American Journal of Forensic Medicine and Pathology* vol. 32, no. 2, June 2011, pp. 104–107.

24. Transformations

p. 241. Ovid, *Metamorphoses*, Book XV, line 260.

p. 241. James Hutton, 'Theory of the Earth', *Transactions of the Royal Society of Edinburgh* vol. I, part II, pp. 209–304, plates I and II, published 1788 (paper given 7 March and 4 April 1785).

p. 242. Ovid, *Metamorphoses*, Mary Innes, trans. Book XV, line 831.

List of Illustrations

While every effort has been made to contact copyright-holders of illustrations, the author and publishers would be grateful for information about any illustrations where they have been unable to trace them, and would be glad to make amendments in further editions.

Index

The suffix 'n' indicates that only a footnote on that page relates to the index entry.